Horse-Sense
Nutrition

Horse-Sense
Nutrition
Fat Loss for Humans

Let's reclaim our innate beauty, health, fitness, and lean body composition.

Carl 6/12

Carl Blake

authorHOUSE®

AuthorHouse™
1663 Liberty Drive
Bloomington, IN 47403
www.authorhouse.com
Phone: 1-800-839-8640

Published by AuthorHouse   Feb. 2012

ISBN: 978-1-4685-3866-3 (sc)
ISBN: 978-1-4685-3812-0 (hc)
ISBN: 978-1-4685-3865-6 (e)

Library of Congress Control Number: 2012900515

Any people depicted in stock imagery provided by Thinkstock are models, and such images are being used for illustrative purposes only.
Certain stock imagery © Thinkstock.

This book is printed on acid-free paper.

Because of the dynamic nature of the Internet, any web addresses or links contained in this book may have changed since publication and may no longer be valid. The views expressed in this work are solely those of the author and do not necessarily reflect the views of the publisher, and the publisher hereby disclaims any responsibility for them.

The information presented in this manual is in no way intended as medical or nutritional advice or as substitute for life coaching. The information should be used in conjunction with the guidance and care of a health professional. Always consult a physician before beginning any program involving diet and exercise.

The author of this book is knowledgeable regarding nutrition, exercise, and stress management but is not a trained professional in these specializations. Consult field professionals before implementing any ideas or practices suggested in this book. The bibliography lists the ample sources that were used as basis for this book written by one layperson for the benefit of another.

Contents

Preface

The best thing that has come along since sliced bread is the idea of not eating it.

"Liberation from the tyranny of excess fat" is the overarching theme of this book. It signifies a process of physical transformation, not a state of being, that continually strives for superior health and fitness. "How will this liberation or transformation occur?" you might ask. It happens miraculously by the body redesigning itself for lean composition as it exchanges fatness for fitness. The human body is a miracle of creation with its highly complex, well-integrated physiological and neural systems evolving over millions of years for ultra-efficiency. Fat metabolism is self-regulating according to five primal functions: to store fat to perpetuate human species by ensuring survival of the individual; to provide energy for normal metabolic functioning; to store waste products that are too acidic and toxic to be circulating in the blood; to supply material for constructing cell membranes; and to carry fat-soluble nutrients. Fat is the body's preferred source of stored energy because it fulfills the body's number one priority of supplying nutrient material to drive all of its biochemical functions. Our bodies were designed to store fat more efficiently than to release it due to environments of unpredictable food supply in which we evolved until recent times. In environments of harsh climate, winter, drought, famine, natural calamity, and predatory co-habitants, our bodies developed energy, stress, and appetite-controlling mechanisms that urged us to hunt, gather, fish, eat, drink, and snack whenever food opportunities presented themselves. These environments no longer exist yet the powerful energy controlling mechanisms in human guts, brains, and fat tissue remain remarkably unchanged from our primal ancestors. In fact, environments in modern industrial countries are antithetical to those which human genes and biology adapted to throughout millions of years of natural selection. This fundamental discord between modern environment of superabundance and primal human biology genetically adapted to uncertainty and hardship is the basis of the modern epidemic of obesity.

Many of us have amassed enough stored fat for decades of winters. We are, in fact, living winters of discontent because fat-shedding springs never arrive. It is time to shed our winters of fat and to live a lifestyle that discourages the accumulation of new fat. Lean body composition, the supreme goal of fat-loss strategy, frees you from insidious cycles of seasonal fat-gain and serial dieting. This lofty goal is in reality the inheritance we can reclaim by surrendering to the supreme power of our cells and genes to mastermind energy consumption, production and expenditure. Our job is easy: to relax and create the proper environmental conditions for the cells and genes to do their job. All that we are and do is negotiated at the cellular level.

Horse-Sense Nutrition: Fat Loss for Humans desires to rediscover with you, dear reader, the high purposes of eating, exercising, and easing stress to leverage the power of your cells, genes, and metabolism in effecting fitness and lean body composition. Giving shape and content to your efforts will help manifest results more easily, sometimes effortlessly. We eat to fulfill the body's primal need for energy and nutrients. All other eating is recreational and enjoyable but potentially detrimental. Although exercise increases metabolism, burns calories, and builds lean muscle, it fulfills an even higher purpose of providing access to goods and services of nutrient-rich blood delivered to the body system-wide. Easing stress is an indispensable part of your self-transformative program because the chronic presence of unresolved stress and cortisol stress hormone can easily sabotage the progress gained from eating and exercising right.

Horse-Sense Nutrition: Fat Loss for Humans is meant to be a fun companion as you transform yourself by building muscle, boosting metabolism, and burning fat. Many of the lesson titles were designed to make you think (and smile) as you begin exercising your brain before pursuing more challenging physical exercise for the body. This is appropriate because the brain controls everything. The most challenging exercise, however, will be found in applying requisite restraint, patience, and resolution in achieving personal goals. Remember: never give up on your high resolve despite momentary lapses.

The vast majority of us have been poorly educated about nutrition. Whether the blame lies with parents, teachers, doctors, nutritionists, fitness trainers, and government food pyramids, you are ultimately responsible for your own state of well-being: physical, mental, and moral. It is never too late for self-correction as long as one possesses the first prerequisite for reversing any condition: to be alive still. Whether you want to add more life to your years or more years to your life, you can attain superior health and a shapely, attractive body as one and the same goal worthy of hot pursuit.

I

Liberation from the Tyranny of Fat

Liberation is at hand! In fact, it's in your hand. *Horse-Sense Nutrition: Fat Loss for Humans* is a manual and companion as you traverse your own unique path to physical transformation. The process of freeing yourself from the physical, emotional, medical, and financial burden of excess fat begins to feel like paradise with access to all the wonderful life-affirming foods surrounding you like the Garden of Eden.

Nutrition is concerned with essential and accessory food substances, their quantity and quality, as means for the human body to obtain optimal performance. We study nutrition in order to determine and refine our understanding of best practices to support bodily needs for energy fuel and nutrients. The body, in optimal health, achieves an ideal composition and distribution of constituent elements similar to the following: water 60%, proteins 18%, fats 15%, minerals 4%, carbohydrates 2%, and vitamins less than 1%. A body approaching this ideal is beautiful both in form and function.

Time is the irreducible, non-negotiable essence of our reality. It can be neither accelerated nor decelerated. Lasting results take time. The most important behavior to cultivate in order to achieve permanent fat loss is patience. In a momentary fit of frustration, do not erase all your hard work by quitting. Stay on the path. Fat loss is as meaningful a path work as any other endeavor because it is through the body temple that physicality, creativity, spirituality, and morality are expressed. Develop higher resolve so that, come what may, you will stay committed to that which you know is the right thing to do, measurements be damned.

Long before becoming overweight or obese, you by-passed multiple opportunities for weight gain prevention. As you employ strategies for fat loss intervention, *Horse-Sense Nutrition* heralds good news and (inevitably) bad news. The good news is that you may not be so bad off after all. You have created mischief in your body, and the body has created its own mischief in you as consequence of aging. A few strategic and major changes, that is, remedial homework, promise dramatic results. Plus they are delicious and mostly easy to implement. The bad news is that you need to get busy starting right now. Like compound interest, investing small deposits as early as possible over extended time yields exponential results. That's why we say, "Time is money." Within a year, you will be able to quip, "Time is lean." Lost time, however, is irretrievable. The battle of the bulge has to be fought on many fronts: muscle loss, physical inactivity, overconsumption, inflammation, acidity, and insulin resistance being the major ones. So grab a glass of water or wine and a fork and let's get started.

This book will momentarily discuss the following points and more:

- Food choices matter. Not all dietary fats are equal. Not all carbohydrates are equal. Not all proteins are equal.
- Fat is the largest hormonal gland of the body and, like muscle, fat is active tissue.
- Rolls of fat aren't attractive, but fat roles are. Admire fat assets.
- Hormones are the power brokers of fat loss. Insulin is the master hormone of fat storage. Unless you are consciously harnessing the power of the hormones for benefit, you are only tinkering around the edges of the fat loss process.
- Exercise has the capacity to transform or recapture the body's efficiency as a natural fat-burning organism. The best form of exercise is the one that you enjoy, perform on a regular basis, and adhere to long term.

- Typical American diets might be deficient in a number of aspects, but dietary protein intake isn't one of them, not even for vegetarians.
- You are not weak and lacking in willpower, just too responsive to deep, biological urges that natural selection has programmed in us.
- Modern obesity-supportive marketing strategies tap into these primal urges. Modifying your behavior with lean-supporting strategies is a powerful antidote.
- Consequences of aging impact extraordinarily on fat loss.
- Only a handful of nutrients are classified as "essential," meaning they must be obtained from dietary sources because the body evolved without the ability to self-manufacture them. In actuality, any substance the body needs becomes circumstantially essential.
- Genetic predisposition and lifestyle factors are equally powerful in determining an individual's acquisition, distribution, and management of fat.
- One of the major problems with American diets is overeating for calorie fuel and under-eating for nutritional support.
- Water and micronutrients are chronically absent in many diets, often masking as hunger.
- Chromium is the missing ingredient in fat loss nutrition. This mineral is the spark that ignites sugar (glucose) metabolism.
- Natural plant foods can be consumed in significantly higher volume because they help to prevent and cure disease due to their tonic, medicinal, and therapeutic effects on the human organism.
- Wheat and gluten protein are considered the chief culprits of foods that trigger fat gain especially when combined with refined sugar and high fat in processed foods. Eliminating them

3

is the quickest means for trimming the waistline and elevating your health to superlative form.

- Some of us are raw foodists; others are vegans or vegetarians. Some of us are frugivores; others are omnivores. All of us, however, are heliovores. Without the sun, nothing on this planet would be possible. Sun is the quintessential source of nutrition for all plants and animals.
- Resting metabolism requires more calories than daily physical activity. Apparently it takes more energy to be than to do.
- Steady-state, low-intensity, slow-durational exercise burns calories primarily from fat. Intense, short-durational exercise does not but has even greater impact on fat loss than steady-state conditioning through additional calories burned after exercise and through increased resting metabolism which draws principally from fat stores.
- The plant kingdom contains all nutritive material for human nutrition.
- Human bodies cannot manufacture a handful of nutrients for optimal functioning: vitamin C, omega-3 and-6 essential fatty acids, and eight to ten amino acids. These essential nutrients must be obtained from dietary sources.
- Food nutrients are not active agents. They are digested and broken down into usable constituents (glucose, amino acids, and fatty acids) for appropriation by the body's biochemical processes. Our job is to create the best conditions for nutrient absorption through good food sourcing and meal practices.
- Four types of activity impact positively on calorie burning.
- Body mass index (BMI) is not an assessment of fitness but rather represents an accurate measurement of weight status for the vast majority of the population determined by height-weight ratio. It is a value that associates risk of disease with excess

weight and obesity. BMI can be an inaccurate measurement of weight status for tall people, athletes with highly developed lean muscle mass (since muscle weighs more than fat), elderly people who have lost significant muscle mass, and dieters who replace fat with muscle.

- Free radicals are neighborhood thugs who also have biochemical rights.
- Your own body and home make the best fitness center; your food and kitchen make the best pharmacy.
- Discover fountains of youth in sleep and stress reduction. Both are highly underrated and unappreciated contributors to fat loss, requiring nothing to do or undo.
- Lean muscle yields higher resting metabolism and predisposes one to a higher level of activity.
- Brown (not white) fat burns fat.
- Fat is easy to acquire but difficult to dismiss. A penny of fat prevention is worth a pound of fat cure.
- For any practice or principle advocated in HSN, you will most likely encounter its opposite even expressed herein. Life itself is inherently paradoxical.

My Fat Loss Success Plan

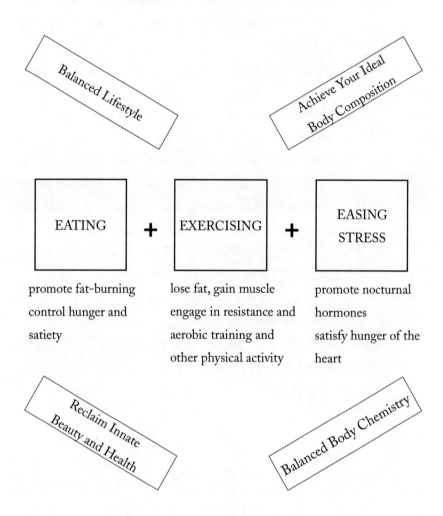

Balanced Lifestyle

Achieve Your Ideal Body Composition

EATING	+	EXERCISING	+	EASING STRESS

promote fat-burning control hunger and satiety

lose fat, gain muscle engage in resistance and aerobic training and other physical activity

promote nocturnal hormones satisfy hunger of the heart

Reclaim Innate Beauty and Health

Balanced Body Chemistry

WHOLE PLANT FOODS NUTRITION

This dietary program supported the human organism throughout
millennia until recent times of food industrialization.
The plant kingdom furnishes the full complexity of essential and
accessory nutrients for humans to survive and thrive.

NUTS ⟶ Nuts and Seeds were the main staple foods of the original
SEEDS ⟶ human diet for reasons of the following:

good source of calories	high unsaturated fat content
good quality protein	minerals and fat-soluble vitamins
fiber	strong antioxidant effects
satiety and pleasure	portability and long term storage
variety of 300+ types	immune-enhancing abilities
blood sugar control	neuro-protective properties
insulin-friendly	metabolic-supportive energy fuel
hormonal balance	plant compounds

VEGETABLES	LEGUMES	ROOTS
FRUITS	STEMS	LEAVES
HERBS	SPICES	FLOWERS
FUNGI	SEA VEGETABLES	CEREAL GRASSES

II

Preliminary Steps for Fat Loss Success
Planetary Nutrients

Step One: Let the Sunshine In

Sunlight enlivens us and improves our health in many ways. No, in every way. Regular exposure to sunshine confers health and beauty by providing denser bones, stronger muscles, healthier nerves, and iron-rich blood. The body has over nine hundred genes with receptors for vitamin D found in brain, muscles, intestines, heart, and blood, demonstrating its key role in overall health: immune, cellular, brain, and cardiovascular health. It builds the immune system and increases oxygenation of the skin. Like magnets, sun and air draw toxic elements in the body to the skin. Sunlight helps regulate insulin by lowering blood sugar. It also aids in storing sugar as glycogen in the liver, muscles, and cells for later use. Sunlight improves eyesight and hormone synthesis. Vitamin D is critical for strong, healthy bone and is necessary to absorb the all-important bone mineral calcium. Vitamin D is *the* superstar fat-soluble vitamin that facilitates cell growth, maintains healthy immune system, and supports blood pressure.

Hear ye, all people who are overweight, dark-skinned, underexposed to sun daily, breast-feeding, or wear sun protection and are dealing with inflammatory problems: you are likely to be deficient in vitamin D, especially D3, the preferred form. The sun is the best source of vitamin D. Everything on the earth is sun-ripened. The sun directly nourishes all. Everything harvests sun energy. Excellent food sources of vitamin D are mushrooms especially chanterelles and pork lard.

Step Two: Air on the Side of Caution

Oxygen is the second-most vital nutrient for life on the earth. Humans breathe seventeen thousand times per day and inhale an average of sixteen thousand quarts of air for our body's sixty thousand miles of blood vessels. Internal mechanisms of breathing are the basis of the evolution of earthly species. Death ensues rapidly without ability to consume oxygen. Although it is hard to believe, we humans consume more air in weight than food and water combined, and we become devitalized when we consume polluted air and water. The best measures for increasing oxygenation of the entire body is being outside and in nature, drinking good quality water, and exercising, primarily walking and participating in more intense aerobic exercise that expands lung capacity. Our ancestral kinfolk were a lucky bunch who oxygenated their brains and bodies with iron-rich blood by walking approximately twelve miles a day. This also maintained their marathoner's bodies. It is believed that this slow, long duration and endurance walking activity provided some extraordinary cognitive or brain-specific benefits: ability to explore and interpret the environment with free hands and active brain, delivery of the body's goods and services enhanced through exercise, formation of new brain cells, and fertile development of healthy brain tissue stimulated by one of the brain's most powerful growth factors, brain-derived neurotrophic factor (BDNF).

Oxygen is a critical chemical element for fat reduction because fat burns only in the presence of oxygen. The more oxygen, the brighter the fire. Keep breathing! It's the most important prerequisite for personal transformation—being alive.

Step Three: Hydration, Liquefy or Dry

> *The human body consists of water for the most part. Nothing better, nothing worse than water—nothing to get excited about. The dry stuff is a mere twenty-five percent of the whole, twenty percent being ordinary egg white, or protein, if you want a little more noble word for it, to which just a little fat and salt is then added. That's about all.*
>
> *The Magic Mountain* (Thomas Mann)

Second to oxygen, water is the most precious element on our planet for sustaining life. Water is the elixir of life. Like the earth, our bodies consist of 70% water with a mineral composition similar to seawater. Water makes up 94% of human blood, 75% of muscles and heart, 83% of kidney and brains, 86% of lungs, 95% percent of eyes, and even 22% of seemingly dry bones. Researchers claim that 75% of Americans are chronically dehydrated, averaging about four glasses a day instead of the generally recommended seven to eight. Dehydration compromises all metabolic systems, nutrient assimilation, elimination of toxins, and fat-burning processes. Hydrating your body responsibly aids cellular processes, energy expenditure and production, and fat burning. Ideal body composition cannot be attained without full hydration, and muscle mass cannot be built without alkalized, oxygenated blood.

The most important first step that *Horse-Sense Nutrition* recommends in accelerating fat loss is to fulfill the daily requirement for replenishing water, the essence of human blood and muscle. The true goal of hydrating the body is not just to satisfy thirst but also to hydrate cells where the most fundamental processes of regeneration take place. Well-hydrated cells speed up cellular renewal as they grow and break down muscle tissue, maintain blood volume, remove toxins and waste products such as carbon dioxide, and promote proper hormone distribution. Food cravings are often the body's desire for water.

Distilled water comes closest to rainwater, once considered the ideal source of water before our atmosphere became so polluted. Bottled water and municipal tap water are generally acidic with high levels of contaminants. Poor quality water can be improved with pH drops or added drops of hydrogen peroxide or choline dioxide. pH drops act as an oxygen catalyst, alkalizing, neutralizing, and oxygenating the body.

Although pure, alkalized, or distilled water is the ideal beverage for humans and animals, other liquids often satisfy thirst and hydrate cells as well, such as water-filled fruits and vegetables that also have high alkaline mineral content. The following are sources of hydration. Some of which are beneficial; others are not. Hydrating sources are not beneficial if they pollute our bodies with any of the following: caffeine, carbon dioxide, chlorinated water, caramel coloring, fake and refined sugars, chemical additives, and aluminum (canned beverages). Raw, freshly pressed vegetable juices that contain leafy greens are highly beneficial. Eating vegetables and fruits and juicing them provide pure, unadultered water filtered through the cells of living plants. Avoid or eliminate pricey energy drinks, because they are highly acid forming and contain toxic levels of caffeine, artificial sugars, colorings, and grossly exaggerated levels of synthetic nutrients and amino acids. It is well to start your day with a glass of water (hot, cold, or tepid) with freshly squeezed lemon juice for internal cleansing and alkalizing body fluids. Drink water and vegetable juices mostly between meals, not with them.

Beneficial Sources of Hydration	Non-beneficial Sources of Dehydration[1]
• water (distilled, alkalized and pure) • extracted vegetable and fruit juices • blended smoothies • water-dense whole fruits and vegetables • raw plant foods • coconut water • herbal and fruit teas • milks • broths • coffee alternatives	• bottled waters • caffeinated energy drinks (diuretics) • alcoholic beverages: wines, beers, hard liquors • canned drinks: sodas, energy drinks • sodium, processed grains, dry foods, and high-temperature cooked foods

Other beneficial practices for occasional use:

- water with dashes of baking soda or salt to alkalize the body
- sensible indulgences including aperitifs (digestive bitters), wine (preferably red), and beer (preferably dark).
- black coffee in small quantities because it is a diuretic, a stimulant, and a highly acidic beverage.

Essential and Accessory Nutrients

Essential nutrients are substances that the human body needs but cannot make itself or in sufficient quantity for optimal health. Dietary sources must provide them. The following chart classifies known essential nutrients critical for good health. All of them are formed first in the plant kingdom.

Essential Fatty Acids	Essential Minerals	Essential Vitamins	Essential Amino Acids
Omega-3 alpha-Linolenic acid (ALA) Omege-6 Linolenic acid (LA)	Calcium Chloride Chromium Cobalt Copper Fluoride Iodine Iron Lithium Magnesium Manganese Molybdenum Nickel Phosphorus Potassium Rubidium Selenium Silicon Sodium Strontium Sulfur Tin Vanadium Zinc	A, retinol and carotene B1, thiamin B12, cobalamin Biotin B2, riboflavin B3, niacin B5, pantothenic acid B6, pyridoxine C, ascorbic acid D, calciferol E, tocopherol Folic acid Inositol K, quinones P, bioflavonoids PABA, para-aminobenozoic acid	Arginine Cysteine Histidine Isoleucine Leucine Lysine Methionine Phenylalanine Threonine Tryptophan Valine

GIVE US THIS DAY OUR DAILY . . .

I. Protein

- Limit total daily intake to 45-80 grams.
- Consume protein in quantities not exceeding 25 grams at any meal, minimally cooked. This amounts to 2-3 ounces or palm-size servings of animal protein.
- Plant sources of protein also count.

WHY? The body recycles proteins and maintains a daily pool of amino acids (proteins) so only a few ounces of protein are needed from time to time to replenish internal supplies. Excess protein whether from total daily intake or individual meal consumption is converted to stored sugar and fat, and promotes cellular proliferation leading to cancer growth rather than cellular repair and maintenance.

II. Carbohydrates

- Emphasize fibrous, nutrient-dense, calorie-sparse, natural whole fruits and vegetables.
- Eliminate or severely restrict as much as possible products of food industry: sodas, sugars, cereal grains, commercial fats, and packaged/processed foods.

WHY? Our diets are too dependent on sugars (natural and manufactured) as primary source of fuel. Thousands of antioxidants and plant compounds residing in natural whole plant foods promote cellular health along with fiber which eliminates cellular waste and prevents its re-absorption.

III. Fats

- Enjoy natural dietary fats—saturated and unsaturated—within reason.

WHY? Fat is extremely important for many cellular and metabolic functions such as protein synthesis and fat metabolism. Fat improves absorption of certain nutrients, makes foods tastier,, and deeply satisfies appetite and hunger.

IV. Nutritional Supplementation

- Supplement, not substitute good dietary habits, with potent substances such as omega-3 oils, multi-vitamin/multi-mineral supplements, and antioxidants.

WHY? The most powerful destroyer of health is oxidative stress to cells and genetic material caused by breathing oxygen, normal metabolism, physical activity, stress, sleep deprivation, toxic environmental pollutants, nutrient deficiency, soil mineral depletion, genetically modified organisms GMOs, sugar indulgence, and contamination of water and food supplies.

RECOMMENDATIONS FOR DAILY FOOD INTAKE

Daily Macronutrients Intake

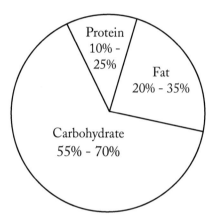

Daily Dietary Fat Intake

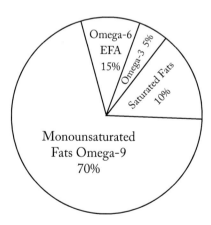

BEST SOURCES OF DIETARY FATS

Monounsaturated	Polyunsaturated Essential Fatty Acids Omega-3s	Polyunsaturated Essential Fatty Acids Omega-6s	Saturated
Omega-9s			
Plant Sources	Plant Sources	Plant Sources	Plant Sources
Avocado + Oil	Flaxseed + Oil	Sunflower Seed + Oil	Coconut Oil/Cream
Macadamia Nut + Oil	Chia (Salba) Seed + Oil	Borage Seed Oil	Palm Oil
Olive + Oil	Canola Oil	Evening Primrose Oil	Palm Kernel Oil
Hempseed + Oil	Walnuts	Black Currant Seed Oil	Cocoa Butter
Nut/Seed Butters	Dark Green Leafy Vegs	Vegetable Oils	
Almond	Hempseed + Oil	Blue-Green Algae	
Peanut		Spirulina	
Pecan		Chlorella	
Cashew		Hempseed + Oil	
Pistachio			
Pumpkin			
Hempseed			
	Animal Sources	Animal Sources	Animal Sources
	Cold-water, Fatty Fish	Egg Yolks	Dairy Products
	Wild Salmon	Animal Meats	Butter
	Sardines	Shellfish	Animal Meats
	Anchovy		Wild Bison
	Mackerel		Beef
	Tuna		Poultry
	Trout		Pork
	Herring		Lamb
	Krill Oil		Animal Fats
	Cod Liver Oil		Beef Tallow
	Wild Salmon Oil		Chicken Fat
	Wild Bison		Lard (Pork)
			Goose Fat

III

Paradigm Shifts in Fork Lifts

This section presents a distillation of some of the simplest and most effective strategies for accelerated yet safe fat loss based on new insights and discoveries by a wide range of disciplines searching for clues in our primal ancestry to promote optimal performance in health and fitness for modern humans. It has come to light that the primal human body of then is essentially the same human body of now. Human survival over the span of millions of years was engineered by the genius of human genetic adaptation. In this age of overindulgent carbohydrate consumption alternating with pernicious low fat diets, we moderns have engineered epidemic obesity and excess weight global-wide. Our only hope for redemption seems to be a return to appropriate human food choices, feeding cycles, native fitness, and circadian rhythms of activity and inactivity for which our primal body and mind were designed by natural selection.

Over recent years, our understanding of fat metabolism has become more enlightened. For example, we have come to respect our bodies as natural fat burning machines because fat is the body's preferred fuel source although it preferentially treats sugar to keep blood sugar levels in check after meals. Weight loss programs are being pushed aside for fat loss programs that specifically target lean body recomposition as the best antidote to fat accumulation. Emphasis on calorie quantity has shifted more to calorie quality, that is, the importance of content and high quality food sourcing. Severe calorie reduction has given way to modest calorie reduction due to research that validates the unintended consequence of significant lean muscle loss that accompanies rapid weight loss. Using mechanical laws of thermodynamics (calories in and calories out) originally applied to steam engines to explain fat gain in humans is losing potency because human bodies are complex biochemical factories and intricate interconnecting information systems not just mechanical machines. Plus, the everyday person cannot with accuracy quantify food calories as we actually eat and metabolize them. Greater awareness recognizes stress as a major cause of weight gain particularly abdominal fat. Fat has only recently been restored to its stellar role as a structural, metabolic, endocrine, and tasty nutritional heavy weight (no pun intended). The true culprits for our predisposition to fatness are carbohydrates especially sugar and wheat, food substances that encourage fat storage due to the massive insulin response they trigger. Excess sugar that is not stored as glycogen in the muscles and liver is converted to fat for storage. Weight-conscious consumers are weaning themselves from dependency on sugar and wheat flour in exchange for fibrous, nutrient-rich vegetables and fruits, natural fats, and quality proteins. Purchase of antioxidant and cellular support supplements surpasses that of expensive exotic fat loss supplements. Short-durational, intense exercise is currently lauded as a superior means of burning calories during and after exercise and for the system-wide benefits it confers on human organism. These and other enlightened notions are leading us out of the woods of fat loss. Momentarily we shall touch on a few everyday practices that keenly impact on fat management: desserts, diets, carbohydrate restriction, meal composition, daily physical activity, exercise, and nutritional supplements.

Ode to Cake (or Joy)

Although it is merely a thick paste that bakes, there is no sorrow that a slice of cake cannot heal. It is one of humankind's greatest creations ranking in importance in human affairs with such inventions as fire, the wheel, steamboats, trains, pianos, electricity, telephones, computers, and iPhones. Ah, cake! You even rhyme with the author's last name: Blake. Such harmonious relations. Nothing seems to slide down the gullet as seductively as cake. Unfortunately, it's the first item that gets deleted from diets except for cheat days. In vain, we hope for a new bestselling diet that classifies cake as a one of the main food groups featured prominently in a revised food pyramid or myplate. Alas, cake eating characterizes one of the most destructive tendencies of modern diets: extreme carbohydrate indulgence with its faustian combination of refined carbohydrates (wheat flour and sugar), protein (eggs), and high fat (butter and milk). Overconsumption of sugars, wheat, grains, processed junk foods, cane and beet sugars, high fructose corn syrup, artificial sweeteners, processed vegetable oils, and stimulants, saps our energy, depresses the brain, and disrupts numerous metabolic pathways. We need to stop thinking longingly about cake as well as finding excuses for its obligatory presence at celebratory occasions. Still, a slice of cake can be enjoyed without self-implosion when usurped as an infrequent use of recreational calories. (See the appendix for a fine cake recipe you can whip up in minutes.)

Cake is not the only culprit. An extraordinary number of other foods are mere variations of cake including: cookies, cupcakes, pancakes, waffles, muffins, donuts, bagels, breakfast cereals, buns, sandwich breads, artisan breads, tortillas, crackers, pastas, candy bars, and snack foods.

Diets, ugh!

All of us have learned by now that diets do not work because the vast majority of them are guises of severe calorie restriction whether they rely on calorie/gram counting or not. Severe calorie restriction is odious to human bodies that are not in tip-top health. Although famine and feast were the norm of hunter-gatherer existence, they no longer are the norm in modern agricultural/industrial societies. Our bodies are programmed to compensate in a number of ways when severe calorie restriction is experienced: the greater the severity of restriction, the more dramatic the compensatory response. Severely restrictive diets increase the desire to eat, cause stress and abdominal fat deposition, decrease physical activity, lower resting metabolism, and degrade lean body mass. Modest calorie reduction, on the other hand, does not evoke these dramatic compensatory responses in the body especially when nutrient-dense foods and small increments of physical activity and exercise are introduced to one's daily regimen.

Our ancestors did not diet, nor did they exercise as activity separate from necessity, nor did they take supplements, nor did they have access to medical technology. They only had their bodies, cells and genes, food, and natural environment to become specimens of athletic prowess. We, moderns, are obsessed with diets. Diets like religion encourage self-righteousness, backsliding, and sinning and promise heaven, hell or purgatory. Leave diets alone. Instead ground yourself in sound nutritional principles.

Carbohydrate Restriction, not Calorie Restriction

For the most rapid gains in fat loss, eliminate or restrict sugars and grains, having no mercy for them or yourself. Since the 19th century, enlightened medical practitioners have noted extreme carbohydrate consumption on the part of people with excess weight. They advocated severe restriction of simple and complex carbohydrates because sugary, starchy, and grain foods have the unique ability to stimulate insulin, the fat storage hormone, and trigger fatty acid synthesis in the liver, a process that floods the bloodstream with triglycerides. Body fat does not burn in the presence of insulin hormone. Wheat and wheat flour, in particular, contain a highly digestible super carbohydrate that is more efficiently converted to blood sugar than nearly all other carbohydrates.

Carbohydrate restriction is also good cancer prevention and intervention. Cancer cells also need nutrition. Recent studies on nutrition and metabolism confirm beneficial effects of a low carbohydrate diet on cancer prevention and treatment. Recent evidence suggests that reducing carbohydrate intake may suppress or delay onset of cancer or cancer growth because malignant cells depend on glucose (blood sugar from carbohydrate metabolism) for energy. High insulin triggered by excess blood glucose also promotes cell proliferation whereas ketone bodies (fat) may not be usable by tumor cells for metabolic demands. Watch your carbs especially wheat and sugar! Try to become as wheat-free and sugar-free as you can stand. If you don't believe that there is life after wheat and sugar, just go to the fresh produce section of your nearest supermarket and introduce yourself.

Ideal Meals as Easy as 1-2-3-4-5

Simplify meal planning by using a feedbag formula that supplies great nutrition and calories for energy. This formula works equally well for all meals: breakfast, lunch, and dinner.

- Drink water or a non-sugared beverage for hydration
- Soup (cup) or Salad (huge volume)
- Protein (your palm-size portion)
- One or two servings of Vegetables (preferably, fibrous, low-sugar, nutrient-dense)
- Healthy Fat added to enhance taste, calories, and satisfaction factor

Remember these actions words of Horse-Sense Nutrition:

CARBS—RESTRICT wheat, grains, sugars, legumes, and dairy
FATS—OIL CHANGE from processed vegetable oils to natural fats
PROTEINS—DON'T overeat or overcook

Repeat after me: RESTRICT, OIL CHANGE, and DON'T!

Foods for Your Feedbag List

- Beverages: water, teas, coconut water, lemon water, and vegetable juices
- Carbs: locally grown or organic fresh produce emphasizing vegetables that grow above ground
- Fats: coconut oil, butter, ghee, lard, and tallow for cooking
- Proteins: wild caught fish, free range chicken and eggs, grass fed or pasture raised meats

Don't forget all the wonderful herbs (fresh and dried) and spices that enhance the taste, digestibility, and presentation of meals. Herbs and spices are amazing nutritional boosts to meals as well.

Condiments are also wonderful taste enhancers: mustard, ketchup (sugar-free), tomato paste, soy and tamari sauce, vinegars, wasabi (horseradish), capers, artichoke hearts, olives, anchovies, peppers (sweet, hot, roasted), nutritional yeast, stevia, honey, syrups, mayonnaise, broths, miso, curry paste, coconut cream, coconut milk, liquid aminos, nuts, nut butters, and flours (almond, hazelnut, coconut).

Snacks are not obligatory but when they are absolutely needed, choose from this list:

- Berries, Whole Fresh Fruits
- Dried Fruits
- Vegetable Juices
- Raw Nuts and Seeds, Raw Nut and Seed Butters
- Soup or Salad
- Protein Shake
- Eggs: hard-boiled or deviled
- Beef Jerky
- Resistant Starch Dishes
- Olives, Avocado (Guacamole), Chunky Salsa, Resistant Starches
- Dark Chocolate
- Leftovers

Increasing Daily Physical Activity

Locomotion (walking and moving around) was the key physical activity that allowed our primal ancestors to achieve daily threshold levels of activity that leveraged our brawn and brain development. In addition to walking an average of 12 miles a day, early ancestors lifted heavy objects, climbed trees, swam, carried objects and children (on backs or in the womb), fought predators and enemies, made tools, played, and sprinted frequently to chase animals for food or be chased by animals for food. Primitive lifestyle required long durational effort drawing on fat stores and short intense bursts of energy that used up sugar stores in the muscles. Protein synthesis rebuilds the body during daily cycles of sleep, anti-stress, rest and recovery after periods of high energy expenditure. On the other hand, modern lifestyle is dominated by chronic stress, sedentary activity, automobiles, public transportation, modern technology, gym memberships, aerobic classes, serial dieting, calorie counting, non-stop feeding, and 24/7 accessibility to food.

Reduction of a mere one hundred calories expended through daily activity can make the difference between gaining or losing ten pounds at the end of a year.

Exercise Benefits

Although increasing physical activity is highly laudable particularly for maintaining weight, more intense forms of exercise are indispensable to serious fat loss. The benefits of exercise have much more far-reaching consequences than calorie burning. Exercise is a tonic to the heart and medicine to our complex organism. Among its benefits, we include the following:

- increases fitness levels which encourage greater energy expenditure during the day
- improves lean body composition which further increases resting metabolic rate as muscle cells require seven times more energy each day than fat cells
- increases fat utilization and decreases fat storage
- increases insulin sensitivity for more rapid and efficient breakdown of fat for fuel
- reverses loss of bone mass
- delivers nutrient-rich blood throughout the body and brain
- helps control appetite
- reduces stress
- promotes longevity largely determined by lean body composition and lung capacity
- reduces risk of injury and onset of diabetes and cancers

Superb Exercise Choices of HIT and Functional Fitness

Exercise researchers have discovered that short, intense interval training is the most effective form of exercise for high-speed fat loss. Why? Because you are burning many times more sugar during exercise and many times more fat after exercise all while doing it in significantly less time. Now you can't beat that even with a stick! Also, this form of exercise is used to treat metabolic syndrome (a common condition exhibiting a collection of symptoms that lead to chronic diseases like diabetes, cancer, and heart disease).

Interval training is easy to implement. Here's how. After warming up for 2-3 minutes, alternate short bouts (20-60 seconds) of intense exertion that creates oxygen debt (signified by panting, gasping, and windedness) with longer intervals (1-2 minutes) of recovery at greatly reduced intensity. During the short, intense bursts you are going for maximal exertion close to 85-90% of your full capacity. When you reach the point where breathing is uncontrollably heavy, you have arrived at your maximal exertion level. (This is the beauty of this exercise form. You don't need a machine with red flashing numbers to tell you when you have arrived at your peak. Your breathing and lung capacity tell you.) During the longer, passive interval, you are exercising at much lower intensity of 30-50% to allow the body to restore the oxygen debt. Repeat five to six sets of these alternating intensities for a total duration of twelve to twenty minutes. On the last set, give it everything you got. DONE! One can perform this type of high intensity workout using aerobic activity (walking, running, sprinting, swimming, stair climbing etc.), exercise machines, weights or body weight. Although many fitness gurus are staunch proponents of HIT (high intensity training) or HITT (or high intensity interval training), Dr. Al Sears' book *P.A.C.E. The 12-Minute Fitness Revolution* is regarded as classic. (PACE stands for Progressively Accelerated Cardiopulmonary Exercise.)

Caution: Do not engage in this form of exercise based on the previously mentioned description. Use caution and research authentic sources, seek professional training, and always consult with your physician before embarking on any exercise or nutritional program especially if you are 50+ years, out-of-shape, carry more than twenty-five excess pounds, or have pre-existing medical conditions. Even when deemed safe to engage in an exercise program, contain your zeal by beginning slowly then progressively increase the intensity over time. Always end exercise sessions with a brief period of cool down (3-5 minutes).

Functional Fitness. Remember high school gym class with Mr. Something-or-Other or Ms. What's-Her-Face? Good old-fashioned calisthenics are excellent exercises for strength training and functional fitness. You remember all those wonderful fitness-enhancing exercises in the halcyon days of youth: jumping jacks, squats, squat thrusts, hand stands, push ups, pull ups, chin ups, sit ups, step ups, dips, rope climbing, sprinting, Supermans, Spidermans etc. How about incorporating these exercises into high intensity interval training to start your mornings, fifteen minutes, three or four times a week right in your own home? That's right. You can turn your home AND EVEN your own body into your favorite gym. Looking for guidance or inspiration? Consult a truly wonderful exercise book by elite trainer Mark Lauren (with Joshua Clark) entitled *You Are Your Own Gym*. It's the bible of bodyweight exercises.

SLEEP

Sleep is every person's private fountain of youth. Sleep deprivation disrupts all the metabolic pathways, increases appetite, causes weight gain especially in the abdominal area (and growing voluptuous breasts on men), and over activates the body's stress response hormone cortisol. Sleeping seven to eight hours each day is the recommendation supported by the medical profession. Turn out the lights and get good, uninterrupted, restorative, blissful sleep.

NUTRITIONAL SUPPLEMENTS

Food and nutritional supplements are a multi-billion dollar industry featuring products that range in effectiveness from miraculous and therapeutic to useless. Of thousands of products available, some of the best researched and processed products are listed below. These nutritional supplements are highly beneficial for lessening the effects of nutrient deficiency of soil and modern food engineering as well as stress, sleep deprivation, pollution, radiation, and environmental toxins. Moreover they detoxify blood and restore integrity to cellular structures. Supplements should be taken according to label directions or as instructed by a medical or nutritional practitioner.

1) Multi-vitamin and Multi-mineral Supplements to address nutrient deficiency and to protect against a gamut of age-related diseases
2) Omega-3's, DHA and EPA Fish Oil to supply essential nutrients that the body itself cannot make, reduce inflammatory response, enhance brain function, improve blood lipid profile, and promote heart health
3) ALCAR or Acetyl L-Carnitine to support brain and nervous systems, fortify vital organ systems, slow the aging of cells, and repair mitochondria (the body's cellular energy factories that also generate free radicals as waste products)
4) Alpha-Lipoic Acid, a super antioxidant, to control inflammation and repair collagen damage

5) N-A-C or N-Acetyl-Cysteine supports insulin function and is precursor to gluthathione (the body's master antioxidant and detoxifier) found in every cell of humans and animals

6) Black Elderberry Juice or Syrup (Berry-Derived Anthocyanidins) to fortify immune defense mechanisms and battle inflammation

IV

Fat Assets

Fat rules! Carbohydrates cannot fulfill the body's tremendous energy fuel demands and protein synthesis cannot take place without the blessings of fat. Though demonized in former decades for their role in epidemics of excess weight and obesity in America, good healthy fats have now been exonerated for their redeeming features and astonishing benefits to fat loss. There are many types of fats or lipids such as sterols (e.g. cholesterol), phospholipids and triglycerides (which comprise 95% of fatty acids in foods and in our bodies). Each type affects the body in a specific way. Fatty acids, the substances which are broken down from fats for body use, bind to specific receptors on cell nuclei and turn on the fat-burning genes in our DNA. The good news for seekers of fat loss is that good healthy fats enhance metabolism, burn fat and promote insulin sensitivity. Fat is indispensable to human biochemistry in a multitude of other functions:

* evolutionary role in survival of human species
* dietary role in brain development in human species
* structural element of cell membranes
* carrier of fat-soluble vitamins A, D, E, and K for absorption in the body
* largest tissue (organ or gland) of the endocrine (hormone) system
* composition of the brain: two-thirds fats
* great determinant of satiety and appetite control
* caloric density two and a half times greater than protein and carbohydrates
* the body's preferred source of stored fuel

- the body's preferred source of fuel for metabolism, sleep, and rest
- protection and cushion for skeleton, muscles, and visceral organs
- primary role in inflammatory processes of the immune system
- constituents of tissues in the heart muscle, sperm, brain, and eyes (especially vital in embryo)
- regulation of body temperature
- endless capacity of the body to convert and store fat for future use
- great taste ingredient

Energy Source Distribution

Sleep and rest are great fat-burning activities. Exercise types draw upon various distributions of energy fuel from fat, glucose/glycogen, and protein. Protein fuel is used very sparingly, not accounting for more than approximately 8 percent in any type of exercise. Low-intensity exercise draws most heavily on fat approximately 65 percent. Light to moderate exercise draws on fat approximately 50 percent. Intense sprinting exercise draws on fat approximately 10 percent and on glucose/glycogen 85 percent. High-intensity endurance exercise draws on fat approximately 40 percent and on glucose/glycogen 65 percent.

Although low-intensity exercise registers a higher percentage of fat use during exercise, high-intensity exercise is also recommended for its ability to burn more fat and more calories during the same period as lower-intensity training and requires additional fat use post-exercise during rest and recovery stimulated by adrenal hormones.

Recommendation of Total Fat Intake

According to the American Dietetic Association, the average person should strive for 20 to 35 percent fat from total daily calories.

For a person requiring two thousand calories daily, this represents 400 to 700 fat calories or 45 to 78 grams.

Horse-Sense Nutrition Guidelines to Fat Assets in Your Diet

- Concentrate on incorporating omega-3 and-6 essential fatty acids (EFAs) throughout the day with particular attention to omega-3 fatty acids: ALA, EPA, and DHA.
- Prefer fats as raw, whole, natural (unprocessed) foods, such as nuts, seeds, fatty fruits, and eggs.
- Enjoy saturated fats and monounsaturated fats in moderation.
- Avoid fake fats such as trans-fats also known as hydrogenated, partially hydrogenated fats.
- Be wary of poorly extracted and contaminated omega supplements.

Excellent Fat Foods

Germinative/ Seminal Foods	Plant Foods	Animal Foods
• flaxseed • chia (Salba) • perilla • hemp • walnuts • whole eggs	• green plants (especially purslane) • avocado • macadamia • canola oil • cereals • breads with nuts and seeds	• fatty fish • wild game • cod liver oil • fish oil • omega-3 enriched eggs • organic dairy products • pastured, grass-fed, or free-range beef, chicken, pork, and lamb

The Skinny on Fat

The comprehensive world of fats is both fascinating and complex. For purposes of everyday nutrition, let's keep fat classifications simple by counting by twos:

- two basic types of fat: saturated and unsaturated
- two types of unsaturated fats: monounsaturated and polyunsaturated
- two types of essential fatty acids (polyunsaturated fats): omega-3 and omega-6
- two types of long-chain omega-3 fatty acids: EPA and DHA
- two types of fake fats: hydrogenated (or partially hydrogenated) and trans fat

Alpha and Omega of Essential Fatty Acids (EFAs)

Does it all seem Greek to you while delving into the nutritional world of EFAs with nomenclature such as alpha, omega, gamma, eicosapentaenoic, and docosahexaenoic? Join the crowd. Even nutritionists have trouble with this topic. Simplicity is key to mastery. Primarily focus on the following fat superstars: omega-3, EPA, DHA, and omega-6.

As miraculous are our bodies are, they cannot manufacture certain essential nutrients critical for normal metabolism, among them vitamin C, a group of amino acids, and two EFAs omega families. Omega-6 fatty acids are found in abundance in many common foods such as nuts, seeds, oils, grains, legumes, and meats. Omega-6s promote healthy skin and support the body's inflammatory responses. Omega-6s convert to both good and bad prostaglandins (hormone-like substances). American diets tend to over-emphasize omega-6 fats.

On the other hand, omega-3s, although represented abundantly in land and sea plant and animal foods, are generally deficient in American diets. The irony of this is that the parent form of omega-3 fatty acids, alpha linolenic acid ALA, is the most abundant fat on earth because it is found in the chloroplasts of green leaves, the most populous foods on the planet. Omega-3 fatty acids are touted for their important role in normal development of the brain, eyes, nerves, and heart. Further, omega-3 fatty acids are critical for brain development in infants. For older people, they serve as good brain foods and anti-inflammatory agents. Omega-3s offer additional great benefits as diverse as protecting the heart from cardiovascular diseases and irregular rhythm, lowering cholesterol, reducing blood clotting, fighting certain cancers, minimizing free-radical damage, boosting immune function, improving memory, restoring mental health, and boosting serotonin and melatonin neurotransmitters. Omega-3s aid weight maintenance and support weight loss efforts through their ability to alter leptin, a hormone that monitors fat levels and supervises hunger and satiety.

Coldwater fatty fish such as wild salmon, tuna, mackerel, sardines, herring, and anchovies are considered superior omega-3 choices with the warning that they most likely contain at least minimal levels of contaminants. Wild bison, grass-fed beef, free-range chicken, and chicken eggs are also considered good dietary choices for EPA and DHA. Animal sources of omega-3 fatty acids are often preferred to plant foods due to the following:

- the rich concentration of pre-formed EPA and DHA fatty acids that they contain in their fats
- the wide range of variability among humans to efficiently convert ALA to EPA and then to DHA

For individuals who prefer purer dietary choices, plant-sourced ALA is recommended with the caveat to increase intake of ALA (the parent form of omega-3) and decrease intake of LA (the parent form of omega-6) since these two acids are metabolic competitors. Achieving a balanced ratio between omega-3 and omega-6, daily intake of 1:4 is considered wiser dietary protocol than preoccupying oneself with absolute quantities of teaspoons and tablespoons.

Canned fish like salmon, sardines, and mackerel, in addition to being ideal omega-3 foods, offer high-quality protein. Canning softens the bones and makes them edible, which provides calcium, fluoride, and phosphorus, essential for maintaining bone health and preventing osteoporosis. Fish oils help improve the ratio between good and bad cholesterol, make the blood less likely to clot, reduce blood pressure, and help prevent irregular heart rhythms.

Eicosapentaenoic acid (EPA) is an offspring of ALA. EPA fatty acids are vital cell messengers and fat messengers. Most animals, including humans, can make EPA from ALA. It is pre-formed in fish, seafood, and fish oils.

Docosahexaenoic acid (DHA), the most abundant fat in the brain, is incorporated in nerve cells and eye tissue. It is an essential factor for brain function, especially cognitive and visual function; nerve cells; and eye tissue as much in infancy as in maturity. DHA is vital for rapid and complex development of the brain prior to and during infancy.

Omega-6 has both a bright and dark side. LA generates derivatives like gamma linoleic acid (GLA), good prostaglandins PG1 and PG3, and bad prostaglandins PG2. (Prostaglandins are hormone-like substances that act as potent cell messengers.) GLA, combined with dietary protein and low-glycemic foods, activates glucagon hormone (the antagonist to insulin) conversion to good prostaglandins PG1 and PG3. Good prostaglandins PG1 and PG3 inhibit insulin release, stabilize blood sugar, increase serotonin production (well-being hormone), provide anti-inflammation and immune function, and stimulate other hormones including growth hormones, pituitary, thyroid, and adrenal. Good prostaglandin production accelerates weight/fat loss and promotes fat-burning metabolism. Excellent sources of GLA are primrose oil, currant oil, borage oil, and spirulina.

Bad prostaglandins PG2 and arachidonic acid (AA), on the other hand, are activated by high-protein or high-glycemic diet, which creates insulin secretion causing fat storage and weight gain. Bad prostaglandins and excess AA contribute to pain and inflammation, constipation, dry skin, depression, skin rash, platelet clumping, and allergies. Oxidation of AA becomes primary fuel for cancer growth in various organs.

Balanced Ratio

It is extremely important to supply the body adequately with EFAs. Striving to obtain a balanced ratio between omega-6 and-3 that approaches the ideal is equally important. Most Americans obtain a ratio of 1:40, ten times too much omega-6! Cut back on omega-6s without eliminating them altogether. They are still essential. The ideal ratio of omega-3 to omega-6 is between 1:1 and 1:4. Rather than worrying about measuring teaspoons and counting grams of essential fatty acids, simply increase intake of omega-3s and reduce intake of omega-6s. As a rule of thumb, all grains are high in omega-6s, and all green plants are high in omega-3s. All oily fish are high in EPA and DHA, and all lean fish are not.

Although omega-6s are abundant in typical American diets, they should not be totally ignored while balancing omega-3s. Excellent sources of omega-6 fats include seeds, nuts, nut and seed oils, vegetables, legumes, and whole grains, for example, the following:

pine nuts	sunflower oil	corn oil	grapeseed oil
pistachio nuts	safflower oil	soybean oil	wheat germ oil
sunflower seeds	vegetable oil	walnut oil	cottonseed oil

Recommendations

- Reduce omega-6 foods such as margarine, salad dressings, mayonnaise, and most fast and processed foods. Increase coldwater fatty fish such as salmon, tuna, sardines, mackerel, and anchovies.
- Aim for 5 to 10 percent of calories from omega-6 fatty acids. Most Americans already get enough omega-6 in foods they are currently eating, such as nuts, cooking oils, and salad dressings.
- Realize that certain foods and food combinations produce greater satiety that others. White meats slim down faster than red due to AA (omega-6 fatty acid) which promotes inflammation and decreases the speed of metabolism. Therefore, increase white meats and lower red meats, but it is not necessary to abandon red meats altogether. Dark poultry is rich in selenium and iron, both useful nutrients for weight loss.

Don't Give Me Flax over Fish

Both plant and animal sources of omega-3 fatty acids are ideal. Omega-3s should be emphasized in the diet. Three types of Omega-3s exist: ALA (the parent form) and its derivatives, EPA and DHA, long-chain omega-3 fatty acids.

Best sources for ALA are plant foods such as algae, purslane, seeds; oils such as flaxseed, salba (chia), perilla and hemp; walnuts; green leafy vegetables; soybeans; and tofu. Fish and animals feed on the ALA parent form of omega-3 to manufacture their EPA and DHA.

The best sources for EPA and DHA are coldwater, fatty fish and fish oils. Smaller amounts can be found in wild bison, pastured or grass-fed beef, and omega-3 enriched eggs.

Flaxseeds are the most abundant source of essential omega-3, making them extremely important for vegetarians because they present a viable alternative to oily fish. Moreover, the benefits of flaxseeds are extraordinary, not to be forsaken in the interest of consuming solely pre-formed omega-3 fatty acids found in fish. Flaxseeds offer both fats and fiber. Fats in flaxseeds thin the blood and, together with fiber, help lower blood cholesterol levels. Fiber in flaxseeds is a good remedy for constipation and helps people with irritable bowel syndrome (IBS). The combination of fats and fiber combats hormone-related cancers, especially of the breast and bowel.

Go Nuts for Seeds

Germinative foods like nuts, seeds, and eggs represent potential life. They have played an important role in human nutrition during millions of years of our existence.

- **Nuts and seeds:** almond, Brazil nut, cashew, chia (salba), coconut, filbert, flaxseed (linseed), hazelnut, macadamia, peanut, pecan, pistachio, pumpkin, soy nut, sunflower, and walnut
- **Nut and seed butters:** almond, cashew, coconut, macadamia, peanut, soy nut, and sunflower seed

Walnuts. Among nuts, walnuts are superstars for the omega-3 fats because they contain levels of serotonin, the mood-altering brain chemical that alleviates depression. Walnuts also contain melatonin, the sleep-regulating chemical that helps people dealing with insomnia.

Fats for Drizzling

Use salad oils sparingly. Learn to enjoy non-oil-based salad dressings by using lemon, Dijon mustard, and fruit. (See appendix for salad dressing ingredients.) Salad oils are flavor enhancers whose fats improve absorption of fat-soluble vitamins A, D, E, and K. Dress up salads to the nines with omega-9s. Monounsaturated fats and oils like avocado, avocado oil, olives, olive oil, and macadamia nuts are great-tasting fats. Other excellent choices include flaxseed, salba (chia), perilla, hemp, macadamia, olive, walnut, and sesame.

Fats for Sizzling

Cooking with fat enhances the taste of meats. In general, fats/oils should be treated like expensive, precious substances to be used sparingly. Challenge yourself always to see how little you can get by with without sacrificing too much taste. The best choices for monounsaturated fats are olive, grapeseed, canola, and avocado. The best choices for saturated fats are coconut oil, butter, ghee, and lard.

Coconut is a medium-chain fat that helps burn fat and is tasty. It is rich in nutrients. Butter enriches cooked and baked foods with its wholesome flavor and texture. Despite bad press and massive misinformation, butter is composed of short-and medium-chain fatty acids that are not stored in adipose tissue but used for quick energy. Fat tissue in humans is mostly composed of longer-chain fatty acids that come from refined carbohydrates. Ghee is better than many other saturated fats. It is flavorful and clean.

Lard is saturated pork fat (extremely popular in the good old days) that has an impressive composition of about 40% saturated, 48% monounsaturated and 12% polyunsaturated fats and a better ratio of omega-3 to-6 than olive, soybean, sunflower, safflower, corn, and sesame oils when it is obtained from truly pastured pigs. Using smaller amounts of saturated fats like lard, butter, ghee, and coconut oil might be better than using larger amounts of polyunsaturated omega-6 fats, both for taste and balanced nutrition. Lard, have mercy!

Need an Oil Change?

Polyunsaturated vegetable oils cause concern due to their molecular instability that makes them prone to rancidity and fast oxidation upon exposure to air, light, heat, and time. They also have an exaggerated ratio of omega-6 to-3.

Perhaps, the time has come to switch to an oil that adds sensational taste and nutritional benefits. Moreover, you can lose unwanted fat by eating more saturated fat in the form of coconut oil and less polyunsaturated fat (for example, extracted vegetable oils). Coconut oil or coconut butter contains medium-chain fatty acids that have fewer calories per gram (6.8 versus 9 calories of other fats). Medium-chain fatty acids do not circulate in the bloodstream like other fats. Rather, they are digested and processed like carbohydrates, directly in the liver, where they are immediately converted into energy. Unlike carbohydrates, however, medium-chain fatty acids will not raise blood sugar. Coconut oil is used for energy fuel rather than fat deposit.

Conjugated linoleic acid (CLA) is saturated fat in animal proteins and dairy products. It has been proven beneficial for fat loss and changing body composition. CLAs are fatty acids from the saturated fats in animal protein foods and dairy products. Tonalin and Clarinol are over-the-counter products featuring CLA. CLA inhibits fat storage in fat cells and stimulates muscle cells to burn fat. A naturally occurring trans fat called trans-vaccenic acid (TVA) is a precursor of CLA and has been proven to help fight diabetes, obesity, and heart disease. (Do not confuse this with trans fat in margarines and fried foods.)

Dietary Cholesterol: A Big Fat Lie

Although the brain is only 2 percent body weight, it hogs 25 percent of the total cholesterol in the body. Cholesterol is required everywhere in the brain and can be appreciated for a variety of purposes as antioxidant, electrical insulator, structural element for the neural network, and functional component of cell membranes. Approximately 80 percent of the body's need for cholesterol is manufactured by cells themselves from saturated fats. Dietary fats make only a small aspect of the body's total need. Even the brain actively uses LDL, the "bad" form of cholesterol. Individuals with low cholesterol levels are considered to be at risk for dementia and Alzheimer's disease.

As an eating and drinking tip, research indicates that red wine reduces post-meal rise of cholesterol. Ten ounces (about two glasses) of red wine after a fatty meal may shield your heart from the meal's adverse effects according to Italian scientists. Less wine may still provide the benefit.

The Reputation of Eggs Made Whole at Last

Recent scientific research has not only exonerated but also championed chicken eggs for the very reasons they were vilified in past decades: peerless protein quality, fat, and cholesterol. Very few foods compete with the nutritional value and versatility of chicken eggs. Eggs contain cholesterol in insufficient quantity to have significant effect on serum (blood) cholesterol. Moreover, eggs are an excellent source of animal protein.

Fear No Fats except Fake Ones

Do not fear saturated fats and cholesterol found in animal foods. They are vital dietary factors necessary for normal growth, proper function of brain and nervous system and protection from disease, and maintenance of optimum energy levels. Almost all fats are mixed with saturated and unsaturated. The basic classification of a fat is determined by its more prominent fat component. For example, even margarine, maligned for being gassed up with hydrogen to obtain a cheap, durable form of fat, contains small amounts of good ol' omega-3 fatty acids. Butter has a balanced ratio of omega-3 and-6 superior to olive oil. Still more mystifying is lard (pork fat), which has a superior omega fatty acid profile than olive oil. Good lardy!

Minimize, avoid, or eliminate fake fats such as trans fat and hydrogenated or partially hydrogenated fats (for example, margarine) as dietary choices because they can actually interfere with the body's ability to metabolize good fats. Hydrogenation pumps hydrogen into fat at extremely high temperatures, changing the molecular structure of fat into trans-fatty acid. Now in a solid form, fake fats have a longer shelf life. Hydrogenated oils tend to promote inflammation. Trans fat stays in the bloodstream for a much longer period of time than other fats and has a harmful effect on cholesterol levels by lowering good HDL cholesterol while rising the bad LDL cholesterol. You do not have to be fanatical about these bad fats. Just make sure that EFAs and other unsaturated fats play a predominant role in your dietary fat.

Cooking Tips for Cutting Fat

One tablespoon of any fat/oil is sufficient to coat the frying pan.
Learn to sauté without oil. Substitute with non-oil substances such
as broth, water, lemon, miso paste, soy sauce, and tea with or without
onions, garlic, herbs, and spices.

V

Supreme Proteins

Second to watery fluids, which constitute 70% of the human body, protein is the second-most abundant substance, constituting 20%. "Protein" is a word that denotes its primal importance in human diet, meaning "of first quality." Proteins are composed of amino acids. Eight to ten of total twenty amino acids in human nutrition cannot be fabricated by the body and therefore must be obtained from dietary sources. These are called essential amino acids. The body cannot use proteins directly. Proteins must be broken down into nitrogen-rich amino acids. Once the digestive system breaks down proteins into amino acids, thousands of proteins are reassembled as building materials for new cell formation and regeneration, neurotransmitters, hormones, enzymes, antibodies, and fuel. A staggering 50,000 proteins exist in the body. These substances perform indispensable biological functions such as the following.

- **Raw materials and building blocks:** new cells, cell regeneration, DNA genetic material, tissues, muscles, blood, skin, hair and nails
- **Neurotransmitters:** messengers for the sensory control center of the brain and nervous system
- **Hormones:** chemical messengers that manage all the metabolic functions of the body
- **Enzymes:** the body's labor force that speeds breakdown and assimilation of nutrients
- **Antibodies:** the body's police force that attacks harmful bacteria and infectious viruses

- **Fuel:** heat conversion during digestion, absorption and chemical changes

Further, protein preserves lean body mass which keeps metabolism efficient.

Protein foods are nutritionally important because they contain the one essential chemical element that fats and carbohydrates lack: nitrogen. Nitrogen is used for creating every muscle in your body and fueling cellular regeneration. Animal flesh foods contain the highest concentration of nitrogen. Plant proteins, though significantly less concentrated, have superior protein quality and greater quantity calorie-for-calorie when compared to animal flesh but have to be consumed in enormous quantities to match even a two-ounce serving of animal flesh. Protein is also important to human nutrition for its high satiety factor, having the ability to satisfy short-term with fullness and long-term with deterrence of hunger.

Protein offers two outstanding weight loss features:

- Protein is calorically cheap because its caloric impact is less than carbs and fats as 25 percent of consumed protein is burned off in heat during digestion, absorption, and chemical changes in the body.
- Protein is metabolically expensive, requiring more calorie energy to maintain than fat.

Inadequate protein intake contributes to loss of lean muscle tissue and, eventually, weight gain, among other serious consequences. Unlike fats and carbs, excess proteins (amino acids) cannot be stored for later use. They must be replenished on a daily basis. Protein, therefore, should be an organizing factor for all meal and snack planning. Determining levels of protein adequacy in daily intake can be problematic and uncertain. Protein deficiency can occur even though adequate amounts are consumed if certain accessory nutrients are missing such as minerals and vitamins (especially vitamin C) for absorption and vitamin B6 (pyridoxine) for transport of essential amino acids.

Nutritionists and medical researchers agree that adequacy of protein intake is one important dietary requirement that almost everyone seems to fulfill whether vegetarian or omnivore. In fact, the true risk might be in the other direction of too much dietary protein intake on a daily basis. Excess of any macronutrient, whether protein, carbohydrate, or fat, converts to glucose (blood sugar) and then fat. In the case of excess protein, the body compensates in two additional ways: urinary excretion of calcium and leaching minerals from bone and tissue to buffer acidity. Moreover, excess protein strains the kidneys. What few professionals don't agree about, however, is the level of adequacy of protein intake on a daily basis. Leaving aside athletes, bodybuilders, and gym rats who have abnormal nutritional needs, it might serve well to identify a general range that characterizes minimal to optimal protein intake for average people. The World Health Organization (WHO), in a 2007 publication entitled *Protein and Amino Acid Requirement in Human Nutrition*, confessed "inherent difficulty" in estimating protein requirements due to questionable reliability of current testing methods. Nevertheless, WHO offered the following guidelines:

- Basal demands (that is, metabolic needs) for dietary protein are quite low, equivalent to 0.3 grams protein/kilogram per day. A person weighing 100 kilograms (220 pounds) would require only 30 grams of protein daily for meeting basal metabolic requirements alone. (Basal metabolism includes all bodily functions just to keep you alive other than your daily physical activity. We shall further discuss basal metabolism in the context of energy imbalance in chapter 7: Primary Causes and Primal Solutions.)

- A total daily protein requirement of 0.66 grams protein/ kilogram per day combining the following addends:

> Essential amino acids 0.18 gram/kilogram + Nonessential amino acids 0.48 grams/kilogram = 0.66 gram/kilogram
> Thus, a person weighing 100 kilograms (220 pounds) would require 66 grams of protein daily for satisfying the mean total protein requirement. This equals a mere 2.5 ounces or a palm-size serving of animal protein.

The recommended dietary intake (RDI of the United States Department of Agriculture suggests 56 grams (minimum) for the average person. Currently, some nutritionists and diet gurus recommend much higher protein intake using multipliers from 0.8 grams to as much as 1.0 grams per kilogram of body weight. Thus, in the case of the same 100-kilogram (220-pound) person, recommendations vary from 56 grams (RDI) to 66 grams (WHO) to 80 grams or 100 grams (various nutritionists and fitness specialists). Age, sex, lean body composition, and level of daily physical activity naturally modify these estimates. Even the highest recommended daily protein intake for our 100-kilogram person, that is, 100 grams daily, would equal only 400 daily calories. Carbohydrates and fats would supply the remaining calories for the day.

A growing number of highly regarded doctors, nutritionists, researchers, raw foodists, vegans, and vegetarians insist that the human body with its highly complex metabolic systems is fully capable of deriving all the essential amino acids from the natural variety of plant foods we encounter in everyday cuisine without having to concoct fastidious meal planning, food combining, and consuming mammoth quantities of plant proteins. All nutritive substances for human nutrition are found in the plant kingdom. Plant proteins are complete in amino acids and do provide us with all the essential amino acids, although some plant foods may be lacking in some or sufficient quantity of all the amino acids. Green plant foods, especially dark, leafy greens, deliver a superior form of protein with additional chlorophyll content that alkalizes the body in addition to the complete array of amino acids.

Protein deficiency is a rarity in American diets, even vegetarian ones. This is partially explained by the fact that protein promotes satiety more efficiently than carbohydrates or fat. It is also partially explained by our culture's obsession and conditioning of animal meat intake.

SUPREME PROTEINS and RAW!

Avocados

Leafy Greens and Juices

Raw Hempnut

Nuts and Seeds

Spirulina and Chorella

Raw Hempnut
Protein Powder

Goji Berry

Edible Wild Plants
(Weeds)

Sprouted Nuts,
Seeds, Legumes

Nut and Seed
Butters

Sea Vegetables

Sprouted Grains and
Grasses

Edamame
(soybean)

Raw Coconut Cream

Raw Chicken
Eggs

Raw Cacao
Powder (Nibs)

Ceviche (marinated
seafood)

Fermented Foods
(Probiotics)

Nutritional Yeast

Raw Wheat Germ

Raw Dairy
Products

Horse-Sense Nutrition Guidelines for Supreme Proteins in Your Diet

Variety of Sources

Protein can be sourced from a wide variety of animals and plants, both land and sea.

Excellent Protein Foods

Animal Flesh	Dairy Products	Protein Concentrates	Green Protein	Sea Vegetables
• wild bison • beef • fish • poultry • pork • lamb • eggs	• yogurt • kefir • hard and soft cheeses • cottage and ricotta cheese	• whey • soy • egg • goat • rice • legumes • nuts • seeds (especially hemp) • whole grains • tofu	• green grasses • dark green, leafy vegetables • sprouts • edamame • wild edible plants	• nori • dulse • kelp • bladderwrack • hijiki • wakame

Source Clean and Lean Protein

Always strive to source protein as wild, pasture-raised, grass-fed, range-free, organic, local, and sustainable. It is better to eat smaller portions of a superior source of meat than larger portions of inferior quality.

Hay, Where Do Horses And Other Animals Get Their Protein?

Believe it or not, protein does not occupy any greater importance or proportion in humans than it does for horses, gorillas, or elephants. Protein for horse nutrition, for example, comes from good-quality pasture and hay. Gorillas, being more closely related to humans, require a more varied diet of fruits, green leaves, nuts, seeds, insects, and dirt bacteria. All nutritive material essential for animal and human nutrition is first formed in the plant kingdom. The biggest concern about protein for human consumption should be quality as opposed to quantity.

Human bodies have free amino acid reserves (the building blocks of protein) circulating in the blood and lymph fluids that contribute about seventy grams of protein daily, from which the liver and cells are continually making withdrawals and deposits. Replenishment of this amino acid pool is not necessary on a daily basis. Nor is it necessary to eat complete proteins at every meal or even every day.

In addition to high-quality protein exemplified in fruits, vegetables, raw nuts and seeds, grains, avocado, coconut meat, and leafy green vegetables, one can add weekly servings of finfish, shellfish, meats, eggs, and dairy products.

Green Is Supreme

The plant kingdom commends the prime sources of utilizable proteins for animal and human nutrition. Dark, leafy greens are nutritional powerhouses offering unparalleled nutritional profiles. They are exceptionally high in antioxidant vitamins A, C, and E and contain over 500 carotenoid antioxidants, flavonoids, and indoles that bind with and neutralize free radicals. Green plants are fiber-rich, which protects from all types of cancers and digestive problems in addition to reducing cholesterol and heart disease.

Take spinach, for example. Just two cups of raw spinach or one cup of cooked spinach yields a treasure trove of micronutrients of RDI (US Department of Agriculture):

Protein	35%	Calcium	25%
Zinc	9%	Magnesium	39%
Copper	16%	Potassium	24%
Manganese	84%	Iron	35%
Selenium	4%	Phosphorus	10%

Popeye wasn't the brightest sailor we've ever known, but he sure knew his spinach. He also picked the right significant other (they never married) in Olive Oyl because some chief vitamins/antioxidants contained in spinach (namely, A, E and K) are fat-soluble.

All preeminent nutritional scholars and researchers recommend that we earnestly consider weaning ourselves from animal flesh-based diets to raw and lightly cooked plant foods, especially green plant foods, as the most effective means for addressing any and all medical concerns, including and especially fat loss.

Don't Be Chicken

Occasionally prefer flyers to fryers. Although one can enjoy chicken, Rock Cornish hens, and turkey in ways *ad infinitum*, one occasionally prefers fowl of a different sort for expanding diversity of fuel and nutrient sources. Try flyers and other fowl such as duck and goose, pheasant, guinea fowl, and grouse from time to time. Poultry meats are high in nutrients. They are a low-fat source of protein (amino acids) and have good levels of B-complex vitamins and minerals. They are energy-rich foods. These nutrients make our nervous system efficient and boost our immune system.

Get Hooked on Fish
(Not Just Canned Tuna and Fish Sticks)

Are you fishing for ways to beef up your meals? Adding variety to routine eating is highly recommended to access the whole complexity of chemical substances vital to superior health. Below is a list of seafood that offers extraordinary health benefits in addition to amazing tastes, textures, shapes, and variety. If you live in coastal areas, many of these marine offerings are imminently available. If not, don't worry. Logistics have made it possible to transport these wonder foods, fresh and frozen, to your locale. How many of these have you tried lately? Vow to extend your life for the next twenty years in order just to get through this list. In fact, becoming a fishmonger will naturally extend your life according to longevity studies.

Nutritional benefits of eating a variety of aquatic species are significant. In addition to being excellent sources of high protein, seafood contains treasuries of vitamins A and E; anti-stress vitamins B (especially B12); minerals such as calcium, selenium, potassium, phosphorus, iron, copper, and zinc; and the brain-boosting nutrients. In addition, fish foods improve blood lipid profile, lower triglycerides, modestly raise HDL (good) cholesterol, help prevent chronic heart diseases, reduce inflammation, and enhance brain function.

All of the following are available seasonally and considered sustainable seafoods, generally free of environmental pollutants and parasites: anchovy, black sea bass, bluefish, bream, butterfish, catfish, clam, cod, crab, crayfish, croaker, John Dory, grouper, halibut, jack, lobster, mackerel, mahimahi, monkfish, mussel, octopus, ono or wahoo, opah, oyster, rockfish, sablefish, salmon, sand dab, sardine, scallop, sea robin, shad, shrimp, skate, smelt, snapper, sole or flounder, squid, striped bass, sturgeon, swordfish, tilapia, trout or char, tuna, weakfish, whelk or periwinkle, white sea bass, and wreckfish.

How do you cook fish? You can steam, grill, broil, panfry, and marinate (like ceviche). Feel free to suck bones for great taste and chew bones for calcium intake. As the saying goes: "The closer to the bone, the sweeter the meat."

Do It Your Whey

The praises of whey cannot be sung enough. Whey protein is an all-natural high-quality protein derived from milk in the cheese-making process. As fresh whey liquid is highly perishable, it cannot be found today except in its powder form as concentrate, isolate or hydrolyzed or in a combination of those forms. Whey has similar composition to human breast milk and identical amino acid composition to human blood. There is no protein food on the planet that competes with the superior biological value (BV as high as 150) of whey protein. Biological value refers to a protein's amino acid profile, rate of digestibility, and effect on muscle growth. Whey's BV is significantly higher than that of eggs, meat, casein, milk, soy, and fish.

Whey protein powder is not only a matchless source of protein but also a treasure trove of alkaline minerals (especially potassium), vitamins, antioxidants peptides, branched-chain amino acids BCAAs for muscle building, and conjugated linoleic acids (CLA) for fat burning. Whey protein is also commended for its metabolic-supportive, immune-protective, and anti-aging properties. Moreover, it is virtually fat-free and carbohydrate-free. In the sports and fitness world, whey protein is revered for its ability to optimize performance when it is consumed prior to muscle exertion. For centuries Europeans have revered whey as a general health remedy and digestive aid.

Quality whey protein is distinguished by the following properties: grass-fed cow's milk, cold-pressed from raw milk, sweet (native) whey, no chemical additives or added sugar or fructose. Whey protein powder is ideal nutrition after intense exercise because it limits muscle protein breakdown, accelerates lean muscles rebuilding, and restores immune function. Combining whey with simple sugars like fruit helps replenish muscle glycogen stores depleted by intense exercise. Quick-digesting protein plus fast assimilating sugar is an unbeatable nutrient combination for the post exercise recovery drink or meal that initiates the anabolic (muscle rebuilding) activity.

Like Little Miss Muffet, sit on your tuffet (after having exercised hard) and eat your curds and whey.

Eat More Plant Proteins, Less Proteins from Industrial Factory Plants

Plant proteins are superior to animal protein, ounce for ounce. Plant proteins are complete, providing all essential amino acids. When you eat plant protein, your body is enjoying amino acids freshly manufactured by chlorophyll and sunlight. Plant proteins offer first-generation, clean, high-quality proteins, not secondhand complex proteins from animals that eat plants or from animals that eat animals that eat plants.

Raw Hemp

Raw hemp is supreme green protein. The nutritional profile of raw hemp is truly amazing, offering alkaline protein with an excellent essential amino acid structure, ideal ratio of omega-3 and-6 fatty acids, high mineral content (especially magnesium, phosphorus, zinc, manganese, and copper), high fiber, no cholesterol, edestin (dominant protein of human DNA), and albumen (dominant protein in human blood and free radical scavenger). To be honest, raw hemp protein is not the tastiest food you will find because hempseed has a very strong character. Yet it is palatable and goes well blended with nut milks and coconut water. Its outstanding qualities recommend getting used to.

Eggs: You Can't Beat Them

Recent scientific research has not only exonerated but also championed chicken eggs for the very reasons they were vilified in past decades: peerless protein quality, fat, cholesterol, and nutrient density. Very few foods can compete with the nutritional value and versatility of chicken eggs. They are both low calorie and low cost. Eggs are an inexpensive source of high-quality protein. Egg protein demonstrates its superior ability to stimulate cellular growth with its rich store of the complete amino acids. With a protein biological value of 94 of 100, eggs are second in protein quality and efficiency to mother's milk for human nutrition. Eggs can be enjoyed in various forms from raw and scrambled to green eggs (and ham) and quiches. They can be served as substantive fare for breakfast, lunch, dinner, and snacks. As nutritional powerhouses, chicken eggs are among the few flesh sources of naturally occurring vitamins D and K, which are associated with longevity and cancer protection. Eggs have high contents of choline, a nutrient necessary for brain and nervous system development and cell membrane structure. Eggs also contain lutein and zeaxanthin, two super antioxidants, and vitamins A, E, and B12. Vitamin B12 is necessary for breaking down fat. The fat in egg yolks contains evenly balanced saturated, monounsaturated, and polyunsaturated fatty acids and no carbohydrates. Free-range chicken eggs generally contain some DHA, (long-chain Omega-3 fatty acids).

Numerous clinical studies have been published declaring no compelling evidence linking egg consumption to heart disease risk. Dietary cholesterol in egg yolks (i.e. zero cholesterol in the whites) has little impact on serum (blood) cholesterol and does not cause heart disease. Rather, blame is on stressful lifestyle and a diet high in foods that elicit increased inflammation, hyperglycemia, and oxidative stress that build up arterial plaque and increase risk for heart attack or stroke among many other diseases. Studies also confirm that consuming eggs on a regular basis accelerates fat loss. Eggs are extremely versatile as seen in the following forms: raw, poached, hard-boiled, scrambled, sunny-side, fried, baked (quiche and frittatas), salad, deviled, and desserts (egg custard, angel food cake, and lemon chess pie).

Ruminate on Dairy Products

Cows, goats, sheep, and buffalo produce milk that we can drink or make into other products such as yogurt, kefir, cheeses, and whey. Dairy products are body and bone builders that greatly aid muscle gain and fat loss. Conjugated linoleic acids (CLA) found in dairy foods is good for weight loss. Buttermilk is alkaline. Butter is ideal saturated fat for cooking and baking. Yogurt, kefir, and colostrums are probiotic (fermented) foods that help create beneficial gut flora. Fat and fat-soluble vitamins (A and D) in dairy, along with alkaline minerals such as calcium, magnesium, potassium, and sodium, make dairy products nutrient-dense.

Go Nuts over Seeds

Nuts and seeds are calorie-dense but also nutrient-dense. As germinative foods, they are small wonders loaded with healthful elements. How do I love thee? Let me count the ways:

1. They are plant foods.
2. They contain no cholesterol.
3. They contain Omega-3 and Omega-6 EFAs.
4. They contain healthy mono-and polyunsaturated fats.
5. They make the heart healthy.
6. They contain small amounts of plant sterols (compounds) that lower blood cholesterol.
7. They lower risk of diabetes by keeping blood sugar stable.
8. They contain abundant antioxidants that protect against certain cancers, Alzheimer's disease, gallstones, and osteoporosis.
9. Walnuts are a prime source of melatonin, a neurotransmitter that initiates sleep and improved brain function.
10. They are rich sources of minerals and fiber.
11. They are available in various forms: raw, roasted, toasted, blanched, salted or unsalted, and candied.
12. They last a long time when stored properly.
13. They are excellent snack foods.
14. They can be incorporated in breakfast, lunch, and dinner.
15. They exist as whole form and nut/seed butters.
16. They trigger a satiety peptide PPY which increases metabolic efficiency.

Choose among the more traditional tasty morsels: almond, Brazil nut, cashew, chia (salba), coconut, filbert, flaxseed (linseed), hazelnut, macadamia, peanut, pecan, pistachio, poppy seed, pumpkin, soy nut, sunflower, and walnut.

Feeling the Heat about Meat

Experimental studies suggest that subjecting meats to high heat as in grilling, frying, and oven roasting meats increases the risk for colon cancer. Stewing and poaching are much safer options of meat preparation. During exposure to high heat (ultra-heat), proteins lose structural integrity, reduce digestibility, and create toxic nitrogen waste, all of which creates carcinogenic (cancer-causing) compounds during protein fermentation in the colon. Even carbohydrates and fats subjected to high heat create cancer-causing compounds but less so than protein. Casein protein, as in melted cheese, in particular, is associated with growth of tumors. It is therefore important to follow these recommendations to reduce risk:

- Identify typical meats in your diet that are grilled, fried, and oven roasted such as hamburgers, hot dogs, sausages, grilled meats, barbeque meats, pizza, eggs, melted cheese, fried chicken, oven-roasted meats, and so forth.
- Limit the frequency of eating meats that are grilled, fried, and oven roasted.
- Limit the quantity of meats that are grilled, fried, and oven roasted.
- Limit the time that you subject meats to grilling, frying, or oven roasting.
- Avoid melted cheese.
- Opt for broth to cook, stew, or poach meats.
- Avoid protein powders that are ultra-pasteurized or derived from ultra-heat processes.
- Bulk up on water-soluble fiber to sweep the colon.

Eat resistant starches to feed gut flora (friendly bacteria) and reduce protein fermentation in the colon.

Raw Meat

For raw food purists, there are some flesh foods that can be consumed in the "raw" such as eggs (raw and uncooked) and seafood (sushi and ceviche). Please be advised, however, that consuming raw animal protein might increase your risk for certain food-borne illnesses caused by microorganisms. Children, seniors and people with delicate immune systems should be particularly careful about consuming raw animal food.

VI

Carb Addictions and Additions

Carbohydrates are the body's main source of energy and the preferred fuel for the brain, nervous system, and red blood cells. Vegetables and fruits have been our saviors throughout millennia. Carbohydrate foods offer what protein and fats do not: sprouts, seeds, roots, stems, leaves, flowers, peels, germ, hull, husks, fiber, and thousands of plant chemicals. Carbs display the phenomenal genetic diversity of our amazing planet with offerings harvested from land, sea, field, forest, and desert sun-ripened for immediate consumption.

Carbohydrates are of four types: simple, complex, fibers, and alcohols. Simple carbohydrates (sugars) are readily absorbed into the body, causing very little nutritional stress and requiring very little energy for digestion. Fruits are exemplars *par excellence* of simple sugars. All energy necessary for digesting starches, fats, and animal flesh protein foods depletes the body of vitality. Complex carbohydrates (starches), on the other hand, must convert to simple sugars during digestion before the body appropriates their fuel and nutrients. Vegetables, cereal grasses, and whole grains are exemplars *par excellence* of complex carbohydrates, although many vegetables are low starch. Fibers are indigestible sugars that cleanse and provide nutrients for friendly bacteria in the digestive tract. Alcohol sugars bypass digestion, and the liver immediately processes them. The body makes alcohols as well. Nature is replete in hundreds of simple sugars, sugar complexes, acids, gums, brans, pectins, and saps, some of which—for example, mushrooms—have medicinal, healing properties. Most of us are familiar with some of the most vital sugars for human nutrition such as human breast milk, glucose, fructose, sucrose, lactose, galactose, fucose, mannose, dextrose, and maltose. The greatest proportion of human nutrition on a daily basis consists of carbohydrates.

Although the nutritional kingdom for humans comprehends plants and animals, all nutritive materials necessary for fueling and supporting human life can be found in the plant kingdom. Plants are the most populous life-forms on earth. Mushrooms alone comprise eighty thousand species. Humans, like animals, could survive as long as a green leaf, stem, root, tuber, herb, grass, berry, nut, seed, fruit, or flower could be sourced. Nutrition that humans derive from animals is secondhand plant material or thirdhand plant material when eaten by animals that ate animals that ate plants.

Carbohydrate plants afford sugar energy, vitamins, minerals, chlorophyll, enzymes, amino acids, antioxidants, probiotics (friendly bacteria), and thousands of plant compounds whose numbers continue to grow even as we identify new ones on a daily basis.

Humans extract energy from plants; plants get their energy from the sun. The sun, in fact, is the source of all life on this planet. The sun transfers energy to soil and air. Plants become green through a chemical process called photosynthesis whereby plants capture the sun's energy and lock it into their roots, stems, leaves, seeds, and fruits. Using the power of the sun, plants draw nutrients from the soil and convert inorganic material into life-giving organic substances. The sun's energy is therefore transferred to animals and humans as they digest plants. The sun nourishes all plant and animal life on our planet. All earthly nutrition can be traced back to the sun. All earthly plants and creatures therefore are truly heliovores before being any other kind of—vore. Moreover, plant and animals are chemically related. For example, the chlorophyll of plants and human blood are almost identical with the exception of one mineral, magnesium in chlorophyll and iron (hemoglobin) in blood. The oxygen that animals and humans breathe comes from chlorophyll-rich green plants. The body transforms chlorophyll into hemoglobin, which the body requires to deliver oxygen and other nutrients to the cells. The most nutrient-dense foods of our planet's cornucopia are chlorophyll-rich grasses: wheat, barley, rye, corn, rice, oats, sorghum, millet, and spelt. The sun is truly the earth's superstar, our inexhaustible source of energy.

Plant carbohydrates are critical. Calorie for calorie, plants are superior in quantity and quality of essential nutrients for human nutrition than other foods. Good carbs are the best fuel source for shaping lean muscle and chasing fat. In fact, fat burns in the fire of carbohydrates. In general, one should consume carbohydrates in a form that is as close as possible to its original natural, sun-ripened state. The medical research community has warned against overconsumption of refined carbohydrates and starches since the late nineteenth century but medical doctors have done a poor job in instructing us in this malpractice of eating. Sugar, the primary element of carbohydrates, can be addictive in excess. Excess carbohydrates, refined sugars and refined carbohydrates, heavy starches, breads, pastas, pastries, candies, pure fruit juices, sodas, energy drinks, and junk foods have recently been incriminated for their preponderant role in the epidemic proportions of overweight, obese individuals not only in the Americas but throughout the world as well. As these problematic foods are deleted and minimized from the daily diet, they must be replaced by delicious, nutrient-dense carbohydrate foods, fresh juices, healthy fats, and quality protein, not only for energy calories they provide but also for feeling fullness and satisfaction, which stave off cravings for sweets.

The Ap-peeling Color of Their Skin

The more you enliven your plate and palate with rainbow-colored plant foods, the healthier and leaner you become. In sufficient quantity, these foods crowd out unnecessary refined foods from diets. The easiest guide to maximizing colorful foods in your diet is the sense of sight choosing the full spectrum of rainbow colors from vibrant to pale: purple, red, blue, green, orange, yellow, and white. The primary pigment of a food represents a special class of nutrients that provide protection in plants as well as in humans.

Curative Power of Roots

A humorous message circulating the Internet extols the curative power of plants and castigates the folly of medical practitioners.

The History of Curing Disease

2000 BC Here, eat this root.
1000 BC That root is heathen. Here, say this prayer.
AD 1850 That prayer is superstition. Here, drink this potion.
AD 1940 That potion is snake oil. Here, swallow this pill.
AD 1985 That pill is ineffective. Here, take this antibiotic.
AD 2000 That antibiotic doesn't work anymore. Here, eat this root.

Eight Vital Sugars

The American palette prefers the sweet to all other tastes and avoids as much as possible the bitter that has cleansing and curative properties. Americans consume more than 120 pounds of sugar per capita annually, which amounts to about a half cup of sugar daily from soft drinks, prepared and junk foods, pastries, frozen desserts, and added sugar. These kinds of sugar (mostly white table sugar) are totally unnecessary for human biology. They are merely taste enhancers appealing to the pleasure center of the brain. Other vital, necessary, and healthy sugars combine with proteins and lipids to form, respectively, glycoproteins and glycolipids. These sugar proteins and sugar fats perform widespread critical functions at the cellular level in every living cell. In fact, without these sugars operating as gatekeepers at the surface of cells, cells would not be able to receive hormones as chemical messengers at cell receptor sites. Cells and tissues need to be renewed, replaced, and regenerated continually. The demands of the body could not be met without cell-to-cell communication that vital sugars provide. Their roles include controlling cellular protein synthesis, breaking down glucose with insulin, building muscle, repairing damage, growing muscle, burning fat, lowering blood sugar and triglyceride levels, inhibiting tumor growth, decreasing inflammation, improving food absorption, sharpening memory, elevating mood, and optimizing immune response.

Sugars are known chemically as saccharides. The vital sugars we are interested in promoting here are monosaccharides with names such as glucose, galactose, fucose, mannose, xylose, n-acetylglucosamine, n-acetylgalactosamine, and n-acetylneuraminic acid. They are important for achieving optimal health and well-being, and they derive from a variety of natural sources. Terrains as diverse as the sea, deserts, woods, fields, and humans (breast milk) are represented by them. Consider these foods as super foods. There's no need to buy super-expensive, exotic foods when many of these foods are probably already at hand. Make these foods carb additions, and minimize carb addictions to white table sugar, high fructose corn syrups, and chemical alternatives.

Food with Vital Sugars
(Monosaccharides or Glyconutrients)

Fruits	Fruits with Pectins	Vegetables	Roots	Desert	Woods	Sea
• berries • currants • tomatoes • figs • coconut meat	• apple • pear • guava • orange • grapefruit • lemon • grape	• cabbage • broccoli • spinach • peas • eggplant • green beans	• carrot • turnip • garlic • onion • leek • radish	• aloe vera leaf gel	• medicinal mushrooms (shiitake, maitake, reishi, and coriolus)	• red algae • seaweed • kelp • chitin • shark cartilage

Gum Sugars	Herbs and Spices	Dairy	Flesh Foods	Grains	Brans from Grains	
• guar • carob • larch tree • astralagus	• echinacea • curcumin • cayenne pepper	• whey protein isolate or concentrate	• hen's eggs • cartilage (bovine and shark)	• corn • oats • barley • rice • wheat	• rice • oat • barley • wheat • psyllium	

Cane the Sugars and Beat the Addiction

The bitter truth about sweeteners is that they are addictive and they are considered the major culprits of the growing epidemic of obesity in the modern global community. Refined sugars show up in just about everything packaged or processed.

Humans evolved with a taste for natural sweetness probably due to the fact that sugar is the primary fuel for the body and preferred source of energy for the brain, nervous system, and red blood cells. The negative effects of refined sugars including table sugar, however, are several. In addition to lowering metabolism, refined sugars create mineral deficiency, especially calcium, causing the body to leach precious minerals from bone and muscle storage. Mineral deficiencies, in turn, create many other conditions. Refined sugars slow down secretion of gastric juice, creating digestive imbalance. Digestion of refined sugars causes severe energy imbalances occasioned by extreme blood sugar spikes and crashes. Finally, the drug-like addictive qualities of sweeteners create craving for more of the same substance. Young people especially have become sugar-dependent.

Not all sugars/sweeteners, however, create severe imbalances. Sugars/sweeteners known as slow-release carbohydrates metabolize slower, resulting in longer-lasting energy and less hormonal imbalance. Quick-release sugars/sweeteners, on the other hand, should be avoided or terminated. Non-caloric artificial sugar alternatives affect individuals in different ways and are meant to be used in extremely small quantities.

Avoid quick-release sugars/sweeteners such as high fructose corn syrup (commercial glucose from chemically purified cornstarch), glucose, dextrose, aspartame, sucrose, and table sugar. Moderately use slow-release natural sugars/sweeteners such as fructose (sugar in fruit and a crystalline sugar), oligofructose (a nondigestible fiber), stevia (an herbal sweetener with a mild licorice taste that is twenty-five times sweeter than table sugar), grape and pear juice concentrates, agave nectar, coconut nectar, brown rice syrup, and maple syrup. Blackstrap molasses (unsulphured) is a good source of potassium, calcium, magnesium, and iron. More acceptable non-caloric sugar alternatives that might even benefit weight loss according to some nutrition professionals are Splenda, sucralose, and acesulfame potassium (Acesulfame K).

Sugar substitutes that have been tested and proven absolutely safe sweeteners are stevia and erythritol. Stevia is extracted from leaves of the stevia plant grown in Brazil and Paraguay. It is 200 to 300 times sweeter than table sugar and contains zero calories. If your brand of stevia has a bitter or licorice aftertaste, it means that it was not properly filtered. Switch to another brand in this case. Eurythriol (better known by its commercial name Truvia) is a safe and healthy sugar alcohol that is 15 times sweeter than sugar and also contains zero calories.

Be Frugal with Fruit.

Fruit is quick energy food that appeals to the rewards center of the brain with "sweetness." Fructose, the sugar that fruit contains, by passes the normal digestive process and goes straight to the liver to be metabolized. Since excess fructose consumption can lead to fatty liver, it is recommended to avoid drinking pure fruit juices habitually but instead eat whole fruit in moderation choosing from the following delectable categories: tropical, citrus, sweet, and fatty (avocado and olives). Fruit, however, is ideal food for post-exercise recovery meals combined with some protein to replenish muscle glycogen stores and accelerate protein synthesis.

Oh, Say Can You Sea Vegetables

The darker hues of these magnificent vegetables—green, blue, red, brown, and black—signal the nutritional richness they add to soups, salads, sandwiches, and sushi. Raw sea vegetables are the most nutritionally dense foods on the planet, offering more than ten times the calcium content of cow's milk gram for gram and many times the iron content of red meats. Wild ocean plants are packed with minerals and trace minerals from the ocean's waters whose chemical composition is strikingly similar to water in human bodies. Sea vegetables are alkaline-forming and contain chlorophyll, naturally occurring electrolytes, and iodine that is critical for important operations of the thyroid, one of them being weight management. Cultivate taste for these varieties: dulse, nori, wakame, arame, hijiki, kombu, agar, laver, kelp, and bladderwrack. Klamath blue-green algae, spirulina, red and brown marine algae, and chlorella can be consumed in supplement form. Sea vegetables are excellent additions to diets because they contain EPA and DHA (long-chain omega-3 fatty acids) also found in cold water fatty fish.

Don't Be a Bean Counter

Beans and peas belong to the botanical family of legumes, plants with pods that contain seeds. Eating beans and peas can be part of a healthy diet for normal individuals. For dieters, they are good for chastening fat. Excellent sources of plant protein, beans and peas are also good sources of antioxidants, minerals, trace minerals, and soluble fiber and do not impact blood sugar or insulin levels in any negative manner. Legumes make wonderful healthy snacks and appetizers. The only caveat is to avoid genetically modified soybeans due to possible health risks associated with their consumption.

Legumes include peas, green string beans, lima beans, black beans, kidney beans, pinto beans, navy beans, garbanzo beans (chickpeas), peanuts, blackeye peas, soybeans, tofu, edamame, fava beans, and cow peas. Some nutritionists object to legumes for two major reasons: 1) humans evolved for millions of years without consuming legumes and 2) legumes contain toxic compounds that are considered major contributors to a large number of modern diseases. The dynamic ecology of the human organism and plant kingdom co-evolved equipping the human gut to handle extremely tiny doses of anti-nutrients (discussed below) such as lectins, protease inhibitors, phytates, gluten protein, phytic acid, saponins, tannins, and isoflavones. Some researchers even believe that exposure to various plant compounds appears to produce a low level of toxemia that provides the benefit of activating longevity genes. Moreover, legumes and grains have played integral roles in agrarian cultures for thousands of years.

Anti-Nutrients

Anti-nutrients are toxic (poisonous) compounds that evolved as protective mechanisms in plants to ensure their survival by offering protection from the harmful effects of ultraviolet (UV) radiation from the sun, retarding microbial decay, resisting climate damage, and keeping away hungry insect pests and animal predators (including humans) from eating them into extinction. All plant seeds contain anti-nutrients but some are more troublesome for human digestion than others. Plant foods that represent the greatest dietary threats are grains (especially wheat), legumes, and nightshade vegetable fruits such as potatoes, tomatoes, eggplant, and peppers. Paleo(lithic) Age diets (e.g. also called primal or evolutionary) present convincing arguments for deleting grains and legumes (especially wheat and soybeans) entirely from one's diet because these food substances are considered nutritional bombs containing a wide array of anti-nutrients including lectins, saponins, phytates, phytic acid, protease inhibitors, gluten protein, allergens, raffinose oligosaccharides, and cyanogenetic glycosides. These toxic plant compounds cause intestinal damage, promote inflammation, agitate the immune system, wreak havoc in the digestive organs, and reduce absorption of nutrients including minerals and protein. Anti-nutrients potentially cause leaky gut and chronic low systemic inflammation and increase one's susceptibility to allergies and autoimmunity. Since humans evolved to tolerate low-grade toxins only in small quantity, foods laden with anti-nutrients should be eliminated, avoided or not featured prominently in our diets. Lectins, in particular, have been associated with leptin (hormone) resistance, a pre-diabetic condition linked with obesity. Predigesting grains and legumes through sprouting, soaking, and fermenting significantly reduces anti-nutrients in plant foods. Cooking also partially diminishes effects of anti-nutrients. Food intolerances and sensitivities are caused by heavy reliance on and overexposure to the limited food sources that dominate Western diets, particularly wheat and soy.

Going Against the Grains

Humans, grains, and grass seeds evolved simultaneously. Moreover, our biological constitution evolved over millennia to accept a certain low-level tolerance and immunity to plant anti-nutrients such as gluten, lectins, phytates, and phytic acid that some grains contain. Scientists assert that human dental structure supports grain mastication and our long digestive tract supports slow absorption of the beneficial nutrients that grains provide. Grains are a broad category of food in which we lump, correctly or incorrectly, a number of edible seeds and fruits of ancient plants that belong to the grass family such as wheat, rice, corn, oats, rye, barley, quinoa, millet, buckwheat, amaranth, spelt, kamut, and teff.

Whole grains offer a broad spectrum of nutrients including fiber, B-complex vitamins, vitamin E, minerals, and health-giving plant compounds such as ferulic and caffeic acids, saponins, and lignans. These stellar substances are generally locked up in the germ and bran of grains, which are removed for refined grain products to make "foods of civilization." It is always preferable to eat your grains whole and home-milled. Be wholier than Thou!

The advice of going against the grains should be heeded primarily in regard to refined grains and their products, not whole grains. Refined grains, puffed up in pride, are usually situated centrally in supermarkets and include such items as breakfast cereals, pastries (packaged and bakery fresh), breads, buns, crackers, flours, baked good mixes, white pastas, and snack (junk) foods. These foods are nutritionally barren and addictive, offering nothing but fleeting satisfaction and rapid blood sugar spikes. Worse still, refined grains are usually paired with refined sugars, salt, cheap and rancid vegetable oils, synthetic nutrients, dyes, fillers, and emulsifiers to mention only a few questionable ingredients.

Grass seeds are much better choices for human nutrition than cereal grains. Also referred to as pseudo-grains, these seeds include amaranth, buckwheat, quinoa, and wild rice. Grass seeds are easily digestible, alkaline-forming, and gluten-free. Packed with nutrition, they contain an impressive array of protein (essential amino acids), fatty acids, fiber, minerals and trace minerals, vitamins A, C, E and B-complex, and neurotransmitters. They can also be ground into delicious flours. Grains and grasses proudly representing the Americas, Asia, Europe, the Middle East, and Africa include wheat, corn, rice, millet, barley, oats, rye, sorghum, teff, Job's tears, mesquite, and couscous. Outside Paleo diet camps (i.e. primal, evolutionary diets), whole grains such as wheat berries, barley, oats, brown rice, and sprouted grains are generally considered acceptable and desirable food choices. Food sensitivities, intolerances, and allergens associated with grains (especially wheat) are caused more often by overexposure to certain limited grains than by their absolute presence. Last, one of the glories of America is our native wild rice, the only uncultivated grain that can be purchased commercially. The nutty, sweet flavor of American wild rice should be a more prominent feature in our diet because all great cuisines of the world are based on local, regional foods and native grains.

Put Fiber in Your Character

Fiber is a magic bullet for weight loss. The benefits of fiber are many. It lowers cholesterol levels, controls blood sugar levels, improves sugar metabolism, assists in nutrient absorption, and reduces risk of diseases, especially those of the bowel. There are several types of fiber sugars: celluloses, beta-glucans, gums and mucilages, hemicelluloses, lignans, nondigestible oligosaccharides, pectins, and resistant starches.

For common understanding, fibers are divided into two basic types according to general physiological effects: soluble and insoluble. Soluble fiber lowers cholesterol levels and helps control blood sugar; insoluble fiber maintains regular bowel function and decreases risk of colon cancer. Soluble fiber dissolves in water; insoluble does not. The presence of either or both communicates fullness during digestion, signaling the hunger mechanism to shut off.

Sources of soluble fiber include high-pectin fruits (for example, pears, apples, peaches, and oranges), corn, oat bran, citrus fruits, vegetables (for example, artichokes, shiitake mushrooms, broccoli, carrots, and sweet potatoes), and legumes (for example, dried beans, peas, lentils, and garbanzos). Sources of insoluble fiber include whole wheat, brown rice, whole grain products, most vegetables, popcorn, and sea vegetables.

Fiber is cellulose sugar found in plants. Cellulose is the cell wall of plants that cannot be broken down in the human intestinal tract. Since fiber passes through the system undigested, no fiber calories are digested.

Strive for 25 grams (minimum) of dietary fiber each day, including 15 grams soluble plus 10 grams insoluble. It is estimated that our Paleolithic ancestors consumed as much as 80 grams of fiber per day!

Don't Stiffen Up about Starch

There is good news for many people who stiffen up when they hear the word "starch." Resistant starch is a recent nutritional concept that exonerates certain comfort foods that were once blamed for expanding our waistlines but are currently considered as potential weight loss benefactors. These are slow-burning starch foods. Because they are served underripe, room temperature, cooled, or chilled, they are thermogenic (fat-burning), requiring the body to expend almost as many calories in digesting them than they are worth. Like dietary fiber, resistant starch stays longer in the stomach and "resists" digestion in the small intestine. It has positive effects on cholesterol, blood sugar and insulin levels. It also speeds metabolism and helps satiety hormones to register fullness so you become sated quicker eating less food. Butyrate is another health benefit of resistant starch. It is an anticancer agent produced by natural fermentation in the colon. Resistant starch has barely one calorie per gram, not four, like regular starch. Salads and side dishes using grains, beans, legumes, and tubers served cold (not hot) are examples of resistant starches, for example, cold potato and pasta salads, three-bean salad, bean salsas, lentil and pea spreads, and sushi.

Other examples of resistant starch foods include fruits (avocados and slightly underripe bananas), vegetables (string beans, peas, potatoes, and sweet potatoes), legumes/beans (kidney, navy, adzuki, black, cannellini, pinto, lentils, and chickpeas), and grains (brown, white and wild rice, barley, bulgur, tabouli, couscous, wheat berries, quinoa, and oats).

If you walk into your favorite supermarket, you will find imaginative realizations of the concept of resistant starch. They can be pricey as portions are sold by weight. You will save a great deal of money making your own. May this list stir your own creativity: potato salad, tabouli, red cole slaw, green cole slaw, black bean salad, quinoa salad, three-bean salad, sushi, spring rolls, broccoli slaw, hummus, tortellini salad, pasta salad, sesame noodles, curried chicken salad, tuna pasta salad, grilled chicken pasta salad, black bean salsa, white bean tuscan salad, orzo with spinach pesto, mango salsa, bow tie pasta with pesto, avocado salsa, guacamole, capellini pasta with artichoke and toasted pine nuts.

Form Alliances with Fight-O Chemicals (Phytochemicals)

Phyto means plants. Phytochemicals or phytonutrients are organic compounds found in plants, especially ones with deep colors of purple, red, green, orange, and yellow. Almost daily, new phytochemicals are being identified. They have many different names but perform similar beneficial roles in human biology, whether their effects are nutritional, medicinal, or toxic. Plant compounds incite numerous antioxidant protective processes, modify gene expression, lessen inflammation, dextoxify, alkalize body fluids, retard or prevent aging and chronic diseases, inhibit blood clot formation, incite numerous protective processes, defend against destructive processes, boost immunity, reduce inflammation, champion beneficial bacteria and friendly gut flora, stimulate anti-cancer defenses, promote longevity, ease digestion, maximize nutrient absorption, and oxidize bad cholesterol.

The number of phytonutrients is legion. More than 4,000 plant flavonoids and 600 carotenoids have been identified. Some of these compounds have antioxidant potential 10 times as strong as that of vitamins C and E. Phytochemicals is a generic term that includes: vitamins, minerals, amino acids, fibers, lignans, flavonoids, flavonols, bioflavonoids, antioxidants, catechins, chlorophyll, polyphenols, phenols, terpenoids, anthocyanins, isothiocyanates, carotenoids, organic acids, phytoestrogens, quercetin, volatile oils, glucoinolates, indoles, thiols, and enzymes.

Doting ANTIs

Accessory nutrients mostly found in plant leaves, stems, roots, flowers, chlorophyll, oils, nuts, seeds, berries, herbs, spices, fruits, and vegetables promote superior health and are characterized by the negative prefix "anti," which means "against" or "not." Like loving aunties, they dote on you. Here are some examples: antioxidant, anti-inflammatory, anticarcinogenic, antiparasitic, antibacterial, antiseptic, antifungal, anti-emetic, antimicrobial, antispasmodic, antitumor, antiviral, and anti-ulcerative. The most notable anti—is antioxidant. Antioxidants are literally lifesavers. They attack, stabilize, and neutralize free radicals or undetached, unstable oxygen molecules that cause damage to cells. Damaged cells sabotage tissue, muscles, and organ systems through cell mutation (replication of sick, abnormal cells).

Some powerful antioxidants are internal to the human body, for instance, alpha-lipoic acid, cysteine, and glutathione. Many foods are antioxidant-rich: fruits and vegetables with rainbow colors and especially cruciferous ones. Other powerful antioxidants include alpha-lipoic acid, cysteine, glutathione, vitamins (both fat-and water-soluble), minerals, fat and oils, and herbs and spices.

Develop a diet rich in plant foods for life-supporting enzymatic action: fruits and vegetables, leaves, stems, roots, flowers, chlorophyll, fibers, plant oils, mushrooms, edible weeds, nuts, seeds, berries, herbs, spices, fruits, and vegetables.

Time for Enzymes

Critically important to our health, enzymes are the body's labor force that initiates or accelerates virtually every biochemical reaction that occurs in plants, animals, and the human body. The fundamental role of enzymes as bioactive catalyst is to break down components of proteins, fats, and starches for digestion, assimilation, and metabolism. More than 5000 distinct enzymes have been discovered. The most commonly known include protease, amylase, lipase, cellulase, phytase, pectinase, peptidase, lactase, maltase, glucoamylase, zylanase, beta glucanase, papain, bromelain, invertase, sucrase, hemicellulase, alpha galactosidase, and dipeptidyl peptidase. When you encounter words with the suffix—ase, you are beholding an enzyme.

Enzymes are tiny proteins or amino acids found in plant foods, the most abundant sources being raw foods. Many physicians and medical researchers believe the fundamental cause of many modern medical conditions is depletion of enzymes in our bodies and absence of enzymes in our diets. The total number of enzymes existing in a typical human body is unknown but believed to be astronomical. A single human liver cell, for example, contains as many as one thousand enzymes. Loading your body with food enzymes may help enhance fat and carb utilization for energy.

All of our digestive and metabolic functions including eating, breathing, sleeping, sex, excretion, nutrient absorption, detoxification, cellular growth, blood circulation, immunity, physical activity, and sensory perception are made possible only by the catalytic work of enzymes in plant foods and those already present in internal organs.

Scoring Points with ORAC (Oxygen Radical Absorbance Capacity)

ORAC refers to the potential capacity of protective compounds inherent in foods to absorb free radicals that can cause tremendous oxidative damage to cells and DNA and throughout the entire body. This scale is a scientific measurement developed by the National Institute on Aging and published by the USDA. Although the scale shares useful information, it has limitations: 1) only 277 foods are tested; 2) all testing took place in vitro (test tube or culture dish), not as antioxidants actually function in the human body; and 3) several different ORAC scales currently exist that propose different values and units of measurements. Nevertheless, ORAC is a handy resource for supercharging your daily regimen with knowledge of the relative power of antioxidant-rich foods. The scale has a range that exceeds 300,000. Just for fun, a brief list of foods with impressive ORAC values appears below revealing some interesting surprises. All measurements are half-cup portions unless otherwise noted.

Food	ORAC VALUE	Food	ORAC VALUE
Acai berry	102,700	Pear, dried	9,496
Goji berry	25,300	Plum	6,259
Blueberry	6,552	Prune	6,552
Strawberry	3,577	Artichoke (boiled)	9,416
Cabbage, red	3,145	Lettuce, red leaf	2,380
Sumac	86,800	Flax hull lignans	19,600
Cinnamon, ground tsp	11,147	Sorghum, bran, raw	312,400
Cloves, ground tsp	13,102	Black pepper, ground	1,151
Oregano, dried tsp	8,339	Parsley, dried tsp	3,098
Turmeric, ground tsp	6,637	Olive oil, extra virgin	1,150
Chocolate, baking, unsweetened	49,926	Pecans	17,940
Chocolate, dark	20,823	Walnuts	13,541
Kidney bean, raw	8,459	Popcorn, air-popped	1,743
Lentil, raw	7,282	Tea, green	1,253
Wine, Cabernet	5,034	Pumpernickel bread	1,963
Corn flakes	2,359	Granola w/ raisins, low-fat	2,294

Other foods that are considered antioxidant all-stars include apples, avocados, beans, broccoli, Brussels sprouts, coconut, garlic, ginger, grapes, kale, kiwi, mushrooms, oats, oranges, pomegranate, pumpkin, spinach, sweet potatoes, tomatoes, and turmeric.

Bitter Now Than Later

Herbs and spices serve equally well in culinary and healing arts. Except among natural health practitioners and their initiates, the health-promoting benefits of herbs and spices are generally unknown. Every kitchen that assembles an array of herbs and spices, fresh and dried, is hospitable to visitors from vast, faraway regions of the globe. They are often the missing ingredients in our diets because of their bitter taste. Herbs and spices are bitter foods that promote digestion and vitally support liver function and detoxification. Bitterness, however, is an important taste to acquire and appreciate. Your liver, the most overworked and unappreciated organ of the body, will thank you because herbs and spices promote beneficial liver function, gentle detoxification, and improved digestion. That's why bitters are commended as aperitifs before and after meals.

Like other plants, herbs are concentrated in essential oils, chlorophyll, vitamins, minerals, antioxidants, and flavonoids. They also host numerous compounds that detoxify and protect the liver, the hub of hormonal activity and master organ of more than 500 important biochemical processes. Maintaining good liver function and liver cell integrity is an indispensable factor for enjoying health, longevity, and vitality. Roots, stems, flowers, leaves, weeds, and seeds are also used to detoxify organs, cure maladies, boost immunity, and restore digestive health in addition to be taste enhancers of savory and sweet dishes.

Spices are culinary alchemists that transform dishes from ordinary to extraordinary. Even the aroma of them stimulates our salivary glands in preparation for gustatory delight. Like herbs, spices are low-calorie and score very high on the ORAC scale for their antioxidant power. Historically, spices were valued for their life force and potent antimicrobial properties that aid in food preservation. Their volatile oils improve assimilation and circulation of nutrients to our digestive system.

Herbs and spices make foods and drinks taste delicious. Familiarize yourself with these wonderful condiments while adding your own personal touch to sweet and savory dishes. Include parsley, basil, turmeric, cinnamon, cayenne and red chili peppers, black pepper, ginger, cilantro, rosemary, thyme, dill, lemon verbena, nutmeg, mace, allspice, and clove. Herbs and spices with extremely high antioxidant properties include cinnamon, cloves, basil, cocoa (cacao) powder, oregano, turmeric, parsley, cumin seed, curry powder, and ginger. Dried herbs tend to score significantly higher than fresh ones.

Herbs, spices, roots, stems, leaves, and flowers have been revered throughout the ages in worldwide cultures as powerhouses of medicinal compounds that offer bundles of benefits across a wide spectrum of ailments and diseases. Herbs and spices, in particular, contain as many as hundreds of compounds that function synergistically within themselves and combined with other herbs create manifold benefits. Ginger, for example, contains nearly 500 beneficial compounds that have been well researched. An extraordinary number of constituents in herbs and spices are still waiting to be discovered. Exhibiting the highest scores among foods represented in the ORAC scale, herbs and spices contain chemical constituents whose actions:

- protect DNA (genetic material),
- stimulate glutathione (the body's master antioxidant and detoxifier),
- moderate nitric oxide (a substance associated with the formation and growth of cancer),
- inhibit inflammatory agents and cancer-producing enzymes,
- clean up oxidized fats and free radical damage,
- heal wounds,

- relieve pain,
- protect digestion, and
- provide anti-inflammatory, antioxidant, antitumor, anticancer, antimicrobial, and anti-ulcerative properties.

Some herbs like ginger, feverfew, and skullcap are additionally noteworthy as the richest plant sources of melatonin, a hormone produced by the pineal gland that regulates the sleep process and inhibits cancer-promoting fat enzymes.

Enjoy the Taste of Time:
Aged, Fermented, Probiotic Foods

Probiotics is the more glamorous term for foods that are cultured or fermented intentionally (that is, not just left to rot). Cultured foods satisfy the taste buds for sweet, sour, salty, and bitter, sometimes all at the same time. Every culture produces its own cultured foods. You've probably tasted a few of these nutrient-rich foods on a regular basis, although hundreds of them exist everywhere: dairy products like yogurt, kefir, buttermilk, and cheeses; sauerkraut and its spicy Korean relative kim chee; fun foods like pickles and meat jerky; alcoholic beverages like beer, wine, and mead; and sourdourgh breads and vinegars with their ageless mothers. Other examples hail from throughout the world: dark beer from Germany, green olives from Spain, sake from Japan, tequila from Mexico, cacao powder from Latin America, coffee from Indonesia, vanilla from Madagascar, teas from China, and spices from India. All of these foods and hundreds more are produced through very simple means of submerging food substances in their own innate juices (namely, lactic acids, yeasts, proteins, enzymes, digested sugars, and fibers) and exposing the mixture to friendly bacteria in the air and time.

If possession is nine-tenths of the law, then our planet belongs to bacteria. They were the first form of cellular life on the planet, and they outlive us when we die (and even help decompose us). Whole new generations of bacteria species of them can be reproduced in twenty minutes. Their numbers are improbably exponential. Human intestinal tracts, for example, house about 1,000 trillion bacteria. We are able to live not with but because of microorganisms. One wonders if they inhabit our world or we theirs. Even so-called "bad" bacteria fulfill a beneficial role as gut flora: decaying indigestible matter and stimulating the intestine to excrete it as gas or stool to remove it as soon as possible. Some bacteria die and then resurrect as antioxidant enzymes to neutralize free radicals.

Probiotics are the best form of natural nutritional support because with them our guts reap significantly higher yield of nutrient assimilation and elimination of waste products. Learning to micromanage microorganisms apparently is the way to longevity. All traditional cultures associated with longevity feature probiotic foods centrally in their cuisine. The most important role that probiotics play in human metabolism is their ability to ease digestion in the intestinal tract by rendering proteins, vitamins, minerals, sugars, fats, fibers, enzymes, and phytochemicals beneficial for human absorption. We safely depend on the innate intelligence of probiotic bacteria to communicate with our immune defense systems in response to the presence of invading pathogens with the command of attack-to-kill.

So the next time you reach for a bottle of supplements of whatever sort, consider consuming on a daily basis a more delicious source of nutritional support. The hundred thousands of compounds already present in your digestive tract might need only the presence of probiotics to release them into action. Cultured foods are easy, fun, and cheap to produce in the home kitchen. Time is the most critical ingredient.

The soaring prices of cultured foods in today's marketplace suggest that time, the most critical of probiotic essences, gets costlier by the day.

By the way, probiotics means "for life" as opposed to its opposite antibiotics, meaning "against life." The former are life-promoting food substances. The latter are drugs that kill viruses and infections and leave residual traces in us.

Grape Expectations.

Add "resveratrol" to your nutritional vocabulary because you will encounter it frequently in current nutritional discussions. Red wine has only in recent years received scientific inquiry revealing its extraordinary health benefits although it has been extolled throughout the ages through common knowledge. Resveratrol is a powerful antioxidant found in red and purple grapes, red wine, blueberry wine, peanuts and peanut butter, pistachios, dark chocolate, hops in beer, berries (for example, bilberry, blueberries, cranberries, and lingon berries), and juices (for example, red, purple, and raw cranberry). Antioxidants are compounds that defend plants against extremes of weather, drought, injury, and fungus to increase their chances for survival. In the case of red wines, the antioxidant resveratrol is concentrated in the skins, which are fermented longer than skins for white and rose wines. In fact, red wines such as Cabernet Sauvignon, Pinot Noir, and Merlot contain ten times more resveratrol than white and rose wines. Volumes of medical research have confirmed potential benefits of resveratrol:

- protects against cellular degradation caused by rampant free radical damage (oxidative stress)
- improves various cancers, depression, Alzheimer's and Parkinson's disease, postmenstrual osteoporosis, liver disease, and LDL (bad) cholesterol

- contains a unique blend of bioflavonoids (plant compounds) and probiotics (beneficial bacteria)
- mimics the same effects on genetic DNA and cellular performance as calorie restriction without a change in eating habits. (Calorie restriction is the only scientifically verified means for improving health and extending life span in animals and humans.)
- improves overall health and aids weight loss through antioxidant and anti-inflammatory protection

The last bit of good news is that the antioxidants comprised in resveratrol improve insulin sensitivity by alleviating oxidative stress to cell. Insulin hormone controls the body's ability to absorb and properly use sugar (glucose) circulating in the blood. Insulin insensitivity (resistance) is one of the biggest factors contributing to diabetes, weight gain, and obesity.

If you currently do not imbibe alcohol, it is not recommended that you start. The benefits of plain red grape juice are almost equal to those of red wine except that the sugar (glucose) content of juice is significantly higher than wine. It you currently imbibe, limit yourself to one five-ounce serving as a female and one to two five-ounce servings as a male. For those who prefer enjoying the benefits of resveratrol without drinking either red grape juice or wine, you can snack on any of the resveratrol-rich foods mentioned above or take resveratrol in supplement form.

As an eating and drinking tip, researchers suggest that ten ounces (about two glasses) of red wine consumed after a fatty meal reduces post-meal rise of cholesterol, thus shielding your heart from possible adverse effects of the meal. Less than ten ounces may still provide this benefit. This is truly having your wine and drinking it, too.

Edible Weeds Supply Your Needs for Diversity

The best human diet is the one that is most diverse, containing domesticated and wild plants and animals, land and sea. Capricious names alone are sufficient reason to pique interest in edible plant foods: jack-in-the-box, stinging nettles, cat's ear, sow thistle, shepherd's purse, sheep sorrel, skunk cabbage, dumb cane, and curly dock. Dandelions and purslane are perhaps more familiar examples of edible weeds that should be cultivated rather than systematically mowed and plucked out of lawns and gardens. There's magic in these two castaways. These weeds are nutritional powerhouses, particularly rich in lecithin, antioxidants, mineral salts, trace elements, pectin fiber, protein, amino acids, vitamins, beta-carotene, and, in the case of purslane, omega-3 fatty acids. Like all green plants, dandelions and purslane contain the healing power of chlorophyll. Yet we yank them up from our lawns with annoyance and later purchase from health food stores the self-same nutrients we've just tossed away. Dandelion roots and greens, blended coffee with chicory and dandelion (delicious), and dandelion wine are current superstars in health food stores. Purslane is almost impossible to find. Cultivate your own until we create a market for it.

All edible weeds offer jaw-dropping nutritional profiles featuring richness of fiber, amino acids, omega-3 fatty acids, vitamins A, E, C, and B-complex, calcium, potassium, iron, zinc, copper, manganese, and selenium. Believe it or not, steamed edible weeds make great pizza toppings, especially dandelion, chickweed, malva, lamb's-quarters, miner's lettuce, plantain, and stinging nettles.

Nutritional Supplementation, Not Mega Doses of Synthetic Nutrients

Nutritional supplements are not good substitutes for nutritional adequacy. Only nutritionists and medical professionals should prescribe supplements to people who have genetic or biological dispositions for not being able to obtain, absorb, or metabolize nutrients from original food sources. Swallowing large quantities of isolated manufactured vitamin and mineral nutrients in pill/tablet or liquid form can create more imbalance than what these substances pretend to correct.

Vitamin C is the only nutrient that the body cannot manufacture but is found in abundant supply in plant foods. Vitamin B12, once thought to be of critical concern especially to vegetarians, is stored in the body and does not need to be replenished on a daily basis. It also turns out that most Americans are not protein-deficient, not even vegetarians.

The best protocol for nutritional supplementation is adherence to plant foods due to their genetic diversity, nutrient density, and calorie sparsity and not to products made from dead plants and animals by pharmaceutical laboratories. Vitamins, minerals, fibers, amino acids, fatty acids, antioxidants, phytochemicals, probiotics, and enzymes that plant foods encapsulate work synergistically to provide antioxidant cellular protection, reduce inflammation, alkalize bodily fluids, and promote optimal metabolism and immune function. Mega doses of synthesized substances used in supplements can lead to toxicity and cellular imbalances that do more damage than good. Only Nature provides certain synergistic factors for repair and regeneration whereby the whole is greater than the sum of the parts. This cannot be manufactured.

Nutritional supplementation is easy to manage when you stick to the cornucopia of foods that you know are good for you: rainbow colors of fruits and vegetables, plant and flesh protein, nuts and seeds, legumes, and sprouted grains. Your gut and brain become enthusiastic receiving wide variety and diversity of foods on a daily/weekly basis.

Knee-d Calcium?

Everybody needs it for at least two reasons: weight gain and risk of osteoporosis as we age. Calcium is well documented as a muscle builder, fat burner, and essential element for maintaining bone mass. Plant sources, however, are excellent sources of calcium without the excess phosphorus that comes with animal flesh products, for example, sesame seeds; dark, leafy greens, especially spinach; green vegetables; sea vegetables; and blackstrap molasses. Anchovies, sardines, and small shrimp are good fish sources of calcium.

Most of us reach for animal products, in particular, milk, cheese, and yogurt, for fulfilling daily requirements of calcium. Excess of meat protein and milk actually causes calcium deficiency. The phosphorus level in meat is very high, and the blood must maintain calcium to phosphorus ratio between one to one and one to two. Excess phosphorus makes blood acidic, which requires drawing calcium from teeth and bones to alkalize it. Excess of both phosphorus and calcium causes the body to bind and excrete them in the form of calcium phosphate because the body cannot absorb it. This leads to further calcium depletion and porous bones.

Plants make strong muscles and bones. Look at horses, gorillas, and elephants for proof.

Losing weight can reduce stress on weight-bearing joints. In fact, a one-pound increase in weight translates into a two-to three-pound increase in the overall force on the knees. Being overweight is directly linked to osteoarthritis of the knee. If you currently do not suffer with knee problems but are overweight, losing weight can significantly cut your risk.

Blackstrap molasses, a dark, bittersweet, slow-moving substance extracted from sugarcane, is great for bone health and preventing osteoporosis. Just one tablespoon contains more calcium than a glass of milk, more potassium than most any other food, and boasts B vitamins, magnesium, iron, and copper as well.

Garlic Roots for Vitamin B12

A garlic tooth offers more than protection from vampires' fangs. All meat and savory dishes benefit by adding sautéed or cooked garlic. In addition to adding great taste, it aids in vitamin B12 absorption. Garlic yields a powerful antibiotic allicin and antifungal compound phytoncide and contains enzymes, flavonoids, vitamins B and C, manganese, selenium, calcium, phosphorus, copper, protein, and tryptophan amino acid. Eating raw garlic summons the sulfur-containing phytonutrient allicin to protect against genetic damage that can lead to cancer. In addition to its culinary value, garlic has been prized throughout millennia for medicinal and therapeutic properties in relieving colds, flus, and cardiovascular and fungal disorders. Ancient Egyptians believed that it possessed sacred qualities. It's hard not to develop a crush on this toothy root.

Recreational Calories: Just Desserts

Desserts belong to a category of eating called recreational or discretionary calories because they are nonessential although enjoyable. The most notable attraction of desserts is that they are tempting. Like Oscar Wilde, most of us can "resist everything but temptation itself."

When assessing whether to abandon or succumb to desserts, keep in mind five points:

- A square slice of cake, say, three inches by three inches, contains five hundred calories with twenty-three grams of fat and sixty-five grams of carbohydrates.
- It has been estimated that Americans eat five hundred calories more per day than they did in the 1970s when we were much leaner without today's admonitions of calorie counting and formal exercise. In the good old days, desserts were generally home-baked and eaten on weekends and special occasions. Don't indulge in desserts on a daily basis.
- When indulging, apply the economics law of diminishing returns to culinary experiences, which suggests that even the most delicious food declines in satisfaction with each additional forkful. Stop after savoring a few bites before reaching the point of "dis-utility" (that is, sickness, feeling stuffed, and added inches to your waist).
- If any dessert, upon first bite, does not inspire awe in you, walk away from it. Don't eat it out of obligation. It's not worth the caloric waste (or waist).
- When you struggle to yield not to temptation, recall the whimsical words attributed to Oscar Wilde: "Moderation in all things is a good characteristic, even moderation itself."
- "The banquet is in the first bite" (adage).

Prize-winning, quick-to-assemble dessert temptations offered in the appendix include General Custard's Vanilla Bean Pudding, My-My-My! Sweet Potato Pie, and Raw-raw-raw Chocolate Buttermilk Cake. You don't have to be a master baker to whip up these three "head-shaking" desserts. Each dish contains a secret spice ingredient. Fifteen minutes of preparation time is all you need to whip them up. The oven does the rest.

CARB ADDICTIONS and CARB ADDITIONS

CARB ADDICTIONS – Eat habitually less of these foods.

refined sugars

artificial sweeteners   pure fruit juices

pastries, candies, sweets   designer energy drinks

products with high fructose corn syrup   junk foods   processed cereal grains and pastas

---

CARB ADDITIONS – Eat habitually more of these foods.

5 – 9 daily
servings of plant foods

rainbow colored   dark green leafy
vegetables and fruits   vegetables

whole fruits   cereal grains (grasses)   nuts and seeds

nut and seed butters   legumes   edible weeds   spices

mushrooms   herbs   teas   resistant starches   edible flowers

VII

Exercise to Exorcise Fat

Muscle and fat relate to each other. Highly developed muscle has threefold capacity to utilize fat and carbohydrate energy fuel, reduce blood fats and cholesterol, and promote insulin sensitivity.

Benefits of Exercise

Almost everyone is aware of the multiple benefits that exercise offers in making you stronger, taller, leaner, fitter, faster, healthier, smarter, and more attractive. Additional factors substantially multiply its benefits: flexibility, physical coordination, cognitive performance, memory, hormonal balance, sense of well-being, cardiovascular health, elevated metabolism, good posture, reduced risk for multiple cancers and diseases of aging, efficient digestion, cholesterol control, oxygenated blood, appetite regulation, excretory regularity, and personal esteem. In short, the impact of exercise on the entire organism is comprehensive. One thing that exercise is not particularly good for, however, is burning calories or fat, at least not during exercise.

Exercise is highly beneficial because it provides improved access throughout the entire body to goods and services already present in the body. The extraordinary effects of exercise take place after exercise during phases of rest, recovery, and regeneration or the metabolic phase of building up known as anabolism. The higher purpose of exercise is to stimulate the body's ability to adapt (evolve or improve itself) in order to meet similar future challenges more fitfully. The responsive adaptation that physical challenge stimulates is an evolutionary principle that allowed our species to survive by overcoming vicissitudes of life and environment whenever and wherever they occurred, very often life-threatening. This adaptive principle is fully operative in our organism still today and is responsible for our being able to survive and thrive while facing the challenges of our time.

Specific to fat loss, the main benefit of exercise therefore cannot be attributed primarily to calorie or fat burning alone but more importantly to stimulating powerful processes in the body that promote overall health in general and, in particular, fat burning while inhibiting fat storage. Exercise combined with sensible nutrition of balanced portions of protein, fat, and carbohydrates from primarily natural foodstuffs is a powerful strategy for fat loss. Eating right and exercising right are inseparable fat loss partners.

Exercise can be *aerobic* (steady state cardiopulmonary conditioning) or *anaerobic* (resistance or weight training). Both forms applied separately or combined can potentially offer extraordinary benefits as much to the entire human organism as to lean body composition specifically in the following ways:

- speeds fat burning
- inhibits and retards fat storing
- preserves lean muscle
- expands lung capacity for greater oxygen efficiency
- creates more lean muscle which burns fat as its preferred energy source
- improves bone mineral mass
- provides volume and flow of oxygen-rich blood to the brain and throughout the body
- balances hormones and hormonal sensitivity
- increases insulin sensitivity at site receptors on cell membranes
- increases basal or resting metabolism which burns mostly fat just to stay alive

- mobilizes and metabolizes glycogen (stored sugar reserves) in skeletal muscle throughout the body
- elevates glucagon (fat-burning hormone) to burn stored fat for energy while lowering insulin levels
- triggers the release of human growth hormone (HGH), another powerful fat-burning hormone
- burns additional calorie energy after exercise while the body adapts to oxygen debt created by high-intensity exercise, a process known as excess post-exercise consumption (EPOC)

A comprehensive exercise program would address inherent capacities of the human body in the following aspects:

- postures for core muscles activation, spinal integrity, and flexibility
- resistance training (with weight or bodyweight) for building strength and lean muscle tissue
- cardiopulmonary conditioning for expanding lung capacity and efficient oxygen use (the foremost requirement of all sentient beings), lung power being the primary predictor of health and longevity
- functional fitness for performing regular daily activities with greater ease and efficiency
- endurance training for reclaiming the innate fitness and beauty of our evolutionary past

Exercise Goals

The quickest, most efficient, and reliable means of losing fat permanently is gaining muscle. Your singular goal, therefore, should be building and preserving lean muscle tissue regardless of your sex or age. Increasing lean muscle will automatically decrease fat in two ways:

- lean muscle draws upon its own sugar fuel stored (glycogen) in skeletal muscles and then switches to stored fat as its preferred fuel
- lean muscle increases metabolism because more muscle requires more calorie expenditure, even during rest.

Sixty percent of calories burned during resting metabolism comes from fat with you doing essentially nothing but staying alive. Many fitness experts currently advocate high-intensity interval training using resistance with weight or bodyweight for strategic muscle gain to achieve lasting fat loss versus water loss or weight loss in which lean muscle is lost. Developing even five to ten more pounds of lean muscle effects impressive gains in fat loss for the following reasons:

- Muscle is metabolically active and burns fat during exercise and rest
- muscle uses oxygen efficiently, and fat burns only in the presence of oxygen
- muscle elevates metabolism while during physical activity and at rest
- muscle triggers human growth hormone HGH, which preserves youthful muscularity and decreases fat
- muscle burns its own stored sugar energy before using stored fat
- muscle development causes fat cells to shrink, and
- muscle helps preserve bone mineral mass.

Increments of muscle gain or development sustained over time improve substantially all organ systems, blood and body composition, and general vitality. It's like residual income 24/7. Deposits of lean muscle continue to work for you free even while you are at rest.

Exercise versus Physical Activity

Exercise and physical activity are not synonymous although both burn calories. Formal exercise is planned activity, requiring more or less intense energy expenditure in short bursts or long, sustained ones that challenge the body to a certain level of fatigue as function of duration, frequency, or intensity. Spontaneous, unplanned physical activity, on the other hand, is not formal exercise yet accounts for a respectable amount of calorie burning just through normal everyday movements, for example, getting out of bed, standing up, pacing while talking on phones, doing chores, engaging in hobbies, carrying groceries, walking the dog, and playing with children. This form of physical activity is called non-exercise activity thermogenesis (NEAT). It is a fairly new concept of energy expenditure that researchers believe stokes your metabolism and can burn as much as 10 percent more calories a day. In fact, for many people trying to lose weight, this form of calorie burning might be a better strategy than exercise. For all of us in need of fat loss, any and all options of calorie expenditure should be exercised. The chart below characterizes activities pertinent to formal exercise and non-formal or NEAT activity.

FORMAL EXERCISE	PHYSICAL ACTIVITY and NEAT
Aerobics: walking, sprinting, swimming, biking	household chores, cooking, hobbies,
weight lifting (resistance training)	brisk walking, standing, lawn and car care, playing musical instruments
recreational sports, calisthenics	fidgeting, dog walking, hobbies, dancing, sex

yoga and Pilates, martial arts	garage cleaning, Little League coaching
functional fitness (bodyweight)	picking up small children, giving massages

Exercise programs should focus on elements such as strengthening the core, increasing flexibility, developing strength, speed, and endurance in addition to bulking up with muscle. The body core (all the muscles and skeletal structure involving the trunk and torso) is involved in all exercises. In addition, many other components of your overall physical education strategy to exorcise fat by increasing lean muscle and fat burning should be added one at a time to your program or exercised alternatively.

- self-massage roller (SMR) or self-myofascial release (release of knots or adhesions in deep tissue)
- spinal flexibility (to relieve stiffness and grumpiness)
- functional fitness (five essential human movements of squat, push-up, pull-up, overhead press, and plank)
- mindful movement (yoga, Pilates, Tai Chi, and martial arts)
- aerobic exercise: constant and rhythmic activity of low, moderate or vigorous intensity
- anaerobic exercise: short-duration and high-intensity activity
- explosive exercise: extremely short-duration and very high-intensity activity
- non-exercise activity thermogenesis (NEAT) (spontaneous play, hobbies, chores, standing, sitting, casual movement, and unplanned activity)

Warm Up and Cool Down are the prelude and postlude to formal exercise routines. Although essential, they are often neglected due to time pressures or disinterest. Spending 5 to 15 minutes warming up prepares the body for work by increasing heart rate and blood flow. Warmed muscles contract and relax more responsively and use oxygen more efficiently. Higher temperatures help nerve transmission and metabolism in muscles. Further, warming up reduces pre-workout stiffness, improves fluency of movement, and sharpens mental focus. The number of nerve and muscle fibers and the rate at which they contract improves with warmed muscles. Spending 5-10 minutes cooling down allows elevated heart rate to recover its pre-exercise state and begin the recovery phase of muscle rebuilding. Last, cooling down reduces adrenaline and waste products built up in the blood during exercise and potentially reduces soreness after intense muscle activity.

GUIDELINES ON EXERCISE
by the
American College of Medicine Sports Medicine ACSM

Workout protocols by ACSM, a preeminent source of exercise research, are supported by indisputable scientific evidence. The following presents the most recent update of their conclusions for cardio training, weight (resistance) training, and functional fitness for adults.

Cardio Training

Exercise at least 2 ½ hours of moderate-intensity exercise per week. This requirement can be met by performing 30-60 minutes of moderate-intensity exercise five days per week or 20-60 minutes of vigorous-intensity exercise three days a week.

Weight (Resistance) Training

Train each major muscle group two or three times per week using a variety of exercises and equipment. For each exercise, go for 8-12 repetitions to improve strength and power; 10-15 repetitions to improve strength for middle age and older persons starting exercise; and 15-20 repetitions to improve muscular endurance.

Functional Fitness
(also known as neuromotor or motor skill exercise)

Train two or three days per week for 20-30 minutes per day. This type of training requires balance, agility, coordination, and gait, very important abilities to develop especially for older adults.

Total training time: 5 hours per week

Body Fat Assessments

Both the quality and quantity of the weight you bear matters. The goal for most of us who carry excess fat is to improve our fat-to-muscle ratio. Keeping track of body fat content is important for planning and achieving success. It is much easier to arrive at a destination once you know where you are starting, and have a viable mode of transportation to get there. Combined, these three indicators provide extremely useful information to help implement your strategic plan of fat loss.

- Bathroom Scales indicate total body mass without differentiating between fat-mass and lean muscle mass. (Newer bathroom scales include water and fat composition as well as bone density.)
- Body Mass Index or BMI is a value that correlates height and weight and a person's risk for diseases. It does not measure body fat.
- Body Fat Caliper Testing is perhaps the best indication of body fat for home use. It measures total body by sampling at a representative site (the suprailliac in the abdominal area). From this measure you can determine how much lean mass you body composition represents. Calipers are easy to use, accurate, and cheap ($20) gadgets that can be purchased online from accufitness.com or from fitness/nutrition stores such as GNC.

VIII

Ease Stress or Stress Ease

Normal daily processes and activities expose us to many negatives whose deleterious effects on our physiology make difficult life in general and fat loss in particular. Multiple stressors of civilization, environment, and personal lifestyle unceasingly sabotage our physical well-being and peace of mind. Stress permeates every aspect of our existence: genetic, aging, metabolic, familial, nutritional, social, psychological, intellectual, professional, environmental, and recreational. Perhaps you can add a few more stressors of your own to the long but not exhaustive list below. Each form of stress produces its own waste products, which creates cellular stress, stress at the most fundamental aspect of our being. Many of us are experiencing a number of these stressors all at the same time.

Genetic	Inherited or acquired genetic defects
	free radical damage
	waste products from energy production
	telomere shortening in genes
Biological aging	Cellular degeneration, loss of lean muscle tissue
	bone density, weakened joints
	weight gain
	hormonal imbalance
	insulin resistance or insulin deficiency
	inflammation
	acidity
	dormancy of human growth hormone HGH
	out-of-whack fat regulatory mechanisms
	sleep deprivation
	chronic stress

Metabolic waste products	Digestion, absorption, respiration, elimination, detoxification, energy production and consumption, breakdown of dead proteins
Familial	Relationships/companionship, rivalry, love issues, responsibility, child rearing, finances, support network, death and loss
Nutritional	Overeating, chronic dieting, nutrient deficiency, fiber deficiency, oxidized fats, overabundance of sugar and refined products, fast foods and junk foods, packaged and processed foods, hormone-injected foods, acid/alkaline imbalance, caffeine
Industrial agricultural	Reduction of modern diet to a handful of types of grains (rice, wheat, corn, and soy), industrial processing of foods, soil depletion, artificial drugs, hormones, and pollutants in animal production, plastics and chemicals in food production and packaging, food dyes, flavorings, preservatives, taste enhancers, carbonation
Professional	Career advancement, unemployment, professional development, undesirable/hostile work environment
Social/ lifestyle-related	Obesity-supportive marketing, abundance of food everywhere, lack of physical exercise/movement, tight shoes and clothes, physical exhaustion
Psychological	Anxiety and depression, social stigma of excess fat and obesity, lack of resolution and inner conflict regarding weight loss, eating as a source of comfort, rising crime levels, neighborhood insecurity, road rage, rude public behavior, waiting and standing in lines, death and loss

Intellectual	Utter confusion about causes and solutions for fat loss, media sensationalism, political instability and ineffectiveness governance at all levels
Recreational	Stress from too little physical activity, stress from too much physical activity, nicotine, alcohol
Drug consumption	Over-the-counter, prescribed, and recreational
Financial	Living paycheck to paycheck, uncertainty of national and global economy, rising costs of foods and shrinking value of the dollar, skyrocketing medical and dental insurance and expenses, uninspiring savings, investments, and retirement portfolio
Environmental	Exposure to sun's radiation, auto exhaust fumes, metal detectors, electromagnetism, electronic devices (cell phones, telephones, and hand-held devices), photocopiers, microwave ovens, x-rays, scans, medical exams, pollution, noise pollution, harmful chemicals, waste disposal, nuclear plants, viruses, harmful bacteria, pesticides, and herbicides

Humans evolved with an exquisite, internal mechanism for managing stress. The body's flawless ability to handle crisis and changing vicissitudes of our reality is key to successful survival and perpetuation of our species. The main effect of stress is to alter the body's chemistry through increased cortisol hormone levels accompanied by a switch to a more sensitive nervous system that gives us the ability to escape (flee) or resolve (fight) personal, situational crisis. All forms of stress, whether acute or chronic, elevate cortisol levels. Acute stress is the momentary confrontation of danger and fear, real or perceived, and dissipates upon resolution of crisis. On the other hand, chronic stress (unresolved and prolonged) maintains elevated levels of cortisol. Chronically elevated levels of cortisol production lead to massive problems and vicious cycles difficult to break, including fat gain. Cortisol, a hormone produced by the adrenal glands, stimulates appetite and, in conjunction with adrenaline, increases fatty acids and blood sugar that eventually are stored deep in the abdominal area, the worst place to carry fat from the standpoint of health.

In addition to its paramount role in stress management, cortisol hormone is critically important in regulating and distributing body fat. The consequences of chronically high levels of cortisol in the bloodstream include the following:

- muscle loss, which leads to fat gain
- slower metabolism, which leads to fat gain
- fat accumulation (belly fat), which leads to fat gain
- leptin resistance (increased appetite and cravings), which leads to fat gain
- insulin resistance (high blood sugar), which leads to fat gain
- insufficient melatonin production (sleep-regulating hormone), which leads to sleep deprivation (insomnia) and disruption of the body's natural biological clock, which leads to fat gain

Excess insulin and cortisol hormones in the bloodstream are perhaps the two most important hormones to balance in order to gain victory in permanent fat loss.

If stress has specific chemistry, so does its opposite calm. The spontaneous combustion of stress occurs by engaging in any beneficial form of being or doing that positively alters the brain's chemistry such as meditation, relaxation, spiritual renewal, creative expression, physical movement, leisure activity, laughter, joy, bliss, and play.

Easy Forms of Stress Busting

Consider engaging in any of these forms of stress-busting on a regular basis:

- breathing exercises (stress changes breathing patterns)
- sleep and relaxation
- rest and recovery
- detoxification
- physical exercise (yoga and Pilates)
- satisfying hunger of the heart: meditation, prayer, religion, spirituality, and healing
- recreational: dance (ballroom, disco, tap, hip-hop, zumba, salsa, and country)
- spontaneous play
- creativity and physical activity
- sports (non-professional and little league coaching)
- hobbies (manual and mental dexterity, creativity)
- charity and volunteerism (sharing/spirituality/compassion)

Sleep Deep and Cheap

Experiencing the nocturnal bliss of sleep is one of nature's greatest gifts. There is no other activity that is so highly underappreciated as agent of anti-aging, elixir of regeneration, and mediator of fat loss. Humans spend one-third of their existence sleeping, experiencing the netherworld of their subconscious and supraconscious selves while the body and brain are busy maintaining and restoring themselves without our intervention. Sleep replenishes our energy supply that gets depleted through constant stimulation from mental and physical activity and the bombardment of environmental stress. Sleep deprivation affects many important body functions such as proper hormone secretion and regulation, food digestion and assimilation, and energy production. In particular, the production of the ghrelin is increased due to lack of sleep or poor quality of sleep. This hunger hormone stimulates overeating and makes you gain weight by lowering the amount of calories you burn. Production of leptin, a hunger hormone that suppresses appetite through carbohydrate metabolism, is disrupted by loss of sleep. Another important hormone cortisol is effectively reduced with adequate and refreshing sleep. Cortisol raises blood sugar and insulin levels which causes an increase in fat deposition especially in the belly. Finally, growth hormone responsible for lean, youthful muscle development and fat burning primarily during the first hours of sleep is diminished by lack of sleep. Many physiological changes attributed to the aging process accompanied by decreased production of GH such as weight gain, obesity, high blood sugar levels, and high levels of free fatty acids in the blood can be ameliorated by getting adequate sleep.

Lack of sleep sabotages weight loss by slowing metabolism, decreasing natural fat-burning mechanisms, and increasing appetite. Sleep loss moreover impairs attention, balance, problem-solving, manual coordination, memory, mood, verbal skill, logical reasoning, and safe conduct. Poor sleep hygiene accelerates the aging process and causes potentially harmful physiological changes that can lead to serious illnesses and diseases such as adrenal dysfunction, nervousness, anxiety, depression, cancer, diabetes, obesity, heart disease, and PMS.

By the way, there is nothing wrong with taking a short nap during the day. It turns out that the biological urge for taking naps is universal among planetary creatures.

Horse-Sense Nutrition Recommendations
for EATING, EXERCISING, and EASING STRESS

EATING

good quality water	improve content of calories	amino acids from plant and
monounsaturated fats/oils	nutrient-dense plant foods	animal sources
Omega-3 and 6 fats/oils EFAs	minimize processed foods	

EXERCISING

aerobic conditioning	improves lean body composition	N.E.A.T. non-exercise
weight (resistance) training	maintains muscle and bone mass	physical activity
functional fitness	accelerates metabolic rate	for calorie burning
	provides nutrient-rich blood flow	
	improves insulin sensitivity	

EASING STRESS

sleep (6-8 hours)	balances hormones, adrenaline,	rest and recovery
spirituality	cortisol, melatonin, serotonin	creativity
relaxation techniques		
intellectual stimulus	satisfies hunger of the heart	volunteerism

IX

Primary Causes and Primal Solutions

"We are what we eat" is a nice phrase to repeat.
"We are what we eat, sleep, repeat, secrete, and excrete" is an
expression more complete.

How we became fat willingly and unwittingly is the subject of this chapter. Causative factors of fat gain are complex and multiple: metabolic, genetic, environmental, behavioral, and cultural. Excess fat in turn exacts its own far-reaching toll on the body and mind (not to mention the wallet and self-esteem) through labored breathing, painful joints, heartburn, depression, sexual dysfunction, and the onset of a host of deleterious medical conditions. We, owners of excess fat, have created poor conditions in our internal environment through conscious lifestyle choices and habits: non-stop eating, 24/7 accessibility to food, instant gratification of fast food restaurants, all-you-can eat buffets, bombardment of obesity-supportive marketing, and overindulgence of carbohydrate foods featuring sugar cane and three grains (wheat, rice, and corn). Behavior modification and cultivation of good habits of eating, exercising, and resolving stress are necessary for remediation. Some conditions result, beneath conscious detection, as deteriorating effects of aging, cellular waste, hormonal resistance, metabolic disorder, nutrient deficiency, acidity, inflammation, and hydration.

Efficient fat metabolism relies on optimal functioning of the whole dynamic human organism with its complex, yet well-integrated organ systems. Permanent fat loss creates a tremendous net gain for the whole organism, not just for your waistline and self-esteem. We shall briefly characterize a wide range of plausible circumstances that very likely contribute to excess fat accumulation and offer possible solutions for remediation. In general, we shall always look to the plant kingdom for its inexhaustible supplies of nutritive, medicinal, and therapeutic substances for improving, retarding, and reversing compromised conditions. The pill that many of us dieters will be forced to swallow is that our diets must replace empty calories from foods from factory plants with nutrient dense plants from Mother Nature.

Hormonal Balance or Hormone-Y (harmony) between Gut and Brain

Hormones are power brokers of fat loss. As chemical messengers of the endocrine system, hormones control or subvert hundreds of vital metabolic functions including sleep, stress, appetite, energy production, protein synthesis, and fat metabolism.

The human body is blessed with large families of hormones to care for it: fat hormones, sugar hormones, brain hormones, gut hormones, stress hormones, male hormones, female hormones, metabolic hormones, and human growth hormone, for example. Traditional hormones you already recognize include insulin, cortisol, human growth hormone, serotonin, melatonin, testosterone, estrogen, and progesterone. What you might not know, however, is that all of these hormones produce metabolic effects that impact critically on fat and carbohydrate metabolism and protein synthesis and degradation. Other hormones with significant roles in fat regulation and appetite control are not so familiar, for example, glucagon, leptin, and ghrelin. New families of fat-and appetite-regulating hormones have been recently added to current understanding of the beneficial and detrimental roles hormonal families play in fat cell biology. Some are highly beneficial with difficult-to-pronounce names such as adiponectin, incretins, secretins, amylin, somastatin, cholecystokinin, glucose-independent insulinotropic peptide, and peptide YY. Other hormones detrimental to fat regulation have scary names in code that make you want to hide behind a tree: TNF, IL-6, RELM, MCP-1, Pref-1, and ASP.

Fat or adipose tissue is the largest endocrine organ of the body. Hormones critical to fat regulation are of five types: fat-burning, fat-storing, fat-regulating, fat-loving, or fat-hating. Among the most powerful hormones are those that regulate appetite and satiety (fullness/satisfaction): ghrelin and leptin, respectively. Primary actions that hormones involved in fat cell biology perform are enumerated among the following:

body fat regulation	fat distribution	healthy peripheral fat	
blood sugar regulation	fat metabolism	unhealthy visceral fat	
blood sugar stabilization	appetite	hunger sex hormones	
food metabolism	satiety	cravings	anti-hunger
energy expenditure	hormonal resistance	body weight	food intake
insulin resistance	leptin resistance	new fat cells	inflammation
insulin sensitivity	leptin sensitivity imbalances	disruptions	

Everything we eat and drink provokes a reaction in our body. Food not only has a profound effect on our metabolism but is also intimately tied up with our emotions and hormones. Even prior to tasting and digesting foods, all the five senses (along with the salivary glands) have awakened the appetite, satiety, and pleasure control centers of the brain. Foods can balance and boost as well as decrease and negatively impact on production of hormones. The brain and gut are in constant communication, interpreting and responding to requirements of body metabolism based on detection of food substances traveling through the intestinal tract. Foods convey specific messages to hormones and hormones deliver specific messages to targeted cells and organs. In general, foods that create hormonal imbalance and cause weight problems are excess sugars and refined carbohydrates. Overconsumption of refined carbohydrates puts one at risk for any number of negative outcomes:

- cause weight gain
- require very little energy to digest
- metabolize quickly into sugar energy
- store quickly as fat
- contain very little fiber to slow down digestion, create fullness, or facilitate elimination;
- are deplete of nutrients such as vitamins and minerals
- decrease metabolism with their dyes, preservatives, and toxins accumulated during storage
- overpower with sugar addictive qualities

Carbs are not bad through inherent qualities but rather through their overrepresentation in our diets.

Some hormones operate as antagonistic pairs. Some keep morning schedules; others are nocturnal. Some hormones have dual personalities, being able to assume different roles at different locations. Hormone sensitivity is the ability of hormones to initiate specific cell reactions. The opposite situation, hormone resistance, occurs when hormones do not reach receptor sites on target cells or circulate in the bloodstream in excess.

Insulin and glucagon are two of the most critical hormones responsible for blood sugar stabilization and regulation. A comparison of these two sugar-regulating hormones in their antagonistic roles appears below. You will notice that insulin hormone kicks in immediately after eating whereas glucagon hormone activates during hunger and turns off when hunger is satisfied. You will further notice in the end that exercise unifies and balances these oppositional hormones, promoting at the same time glucagon production and insulin sensitivity, a double whammy benefit for fat management.

Insulin Hormone	Glucagon Hormone
serves to stabilize blood sugar	serves to stabilize blood sugar
produced by beta cells of the pancreas	produced by alpha cells of the pancreas
opposite effect of glucagon hormone	opposite effect of insulin hormone
causes cravings when in excess	abates when hunger is satisfied
promotes weight gain	promotes weight loss
produces fat storage with excess glucose	stimulates stored sugar and fat burning in muscles
increases by frequency of meals	increases during five to six hours of non-eating
releases in presence of excess sugar	increases when food is present in digestive tract
overproduction is highly undesirable	releases when blood glucose level is low
exercise improves insulin sensitivity	exercise promotes glucagon production

The endocrine system maintains an intricate and interconnected hierarchy of hormonal pathways in which insulin hormone tends to dominate, blocking access of competing hormones at cell receptor sites. Excess insulin can even outperform the thyroid's hormones, resulting in lower metabolism.

Overconsumption of natural carbohydrates (simple and complex), refined sugars and grains, and processed foods creates excess sugar (glucose) circulating chronically in the bloodstream, which makes the pancreas overproduce insulin in order to balance blood sugar levels. Insulin resistance and low insulin production create vicious cycles of blood sugar spikes and lows. Further, overproduction of insulin strains and exhausts the pancreas and liver, hubs of hormonal activity. Although carbohydrates (especially refined ones) are almost wholly singled out as culprits for causing excess insulin secretion, it is important to bear in mind that all food macronutrients—proteins and fats as well as carbohydrates—promote insulin secretion. Excess of any food type potentially converts to fat. For example, excess sugar that cannot be used as glucose (blood sugar) is first stored as glycogen in the liver and muscles. Excess sugar that is not stored as glycogen in the liver and muscles is converted to triglycerides to be stored as fat or serum (blood) cholesterol. Elevated insulin levels in the bloodstream contribute mightily to fat storage.

Over time, the combination of exhausted liver and pancreas, insulin resistance, and excess fat accumulation lead to disastrous consequences not only of tremendous weight gain and obesity but also to the onset of pre-diabetes, diabetes, and a host of other medical and psychological maladies including heart disease, various cancers, insomnia, anxiety, and depression. Last, hormonal imbalance accelerates aging at the cellular level and sets you on the path toward serious disease.

Primal Solutions

Harness the power of the hormones to achieve fat loss through simple and effective means including the following:

- Regulating blood sugar with frequent, small, and balanced meals and snacks that combine all three macronutrients: protein, fat, and carbohydrates, that is, mixed meals.
- Avoiding overconsumption at meals or snacks.

- Eliminating or severely restricting refined sugars, refined carbohydrates, sodas, pure fruit juices, junk foods, and desserts.
- Hydrating with water.
- Eating to satiety with large volumes of fibrous, nutrient dense, low-glycemic carbohydrate foods (vegetables and fruits) combined with adequate amounts of quality protein.
- Adding beneficial fats such as nuts, seeds, fish oils, and coconut oil for greater satiety and metabolic efficiency.
- Exercising to improve hormone production and hormone sensitivity.

Foods and Beverages
That Promote Hormonal Balance

- adequate protein including meats, seafoods, poultry, and eggs
- natural fats including saturated and unsaturated
- omega-3 EFAs(fish and fish oils) and monounsaturated fats (olive and avocado oils)
- nuts and seeds
- fruits
- vegetables
- slow-digesting (resistant) carbs
- whole grains
- fiber
- clean water
- green tea
- selenium-rich foods including whole grains, brewer's yeast, vegetables, and fruits

- potassium-rich foods including legumes, fruits, avocados, and vegetables
- zinc-rich foods including seafood, dark meat in poultry, and nuts
- magnesium-rich foods including beans, seeds, and whole grains
- cinnamon and clove (spices turn on your insulin receptors on cell membranes)

Evolutionary Design

Natural selection designed fat as an internal self-regulating mechanism to protect against starvation and promote survival of the individual during lean times, drought, famine, and pregnancy. Alas, this trait is maladaptive in modern environments of super-abundance. Ancestral humans had the capacity to store body fat with ease when opportunities to consume excess calories arose, but food scarcity and high levels of physical activity offset that trait. Modern humans find themselves in obeso-genic environments that are antithetical to environments in which our complex genetic and biological systems evolved. Reduction of heavy manual work, use of labor saving devices and transportation vehicles, and inexhaustible food supplies put us at significantly greater risk for excess stored fat through ease in calorie consumption and diminished energy expenditure.

Genetic Disposition

Genes are responsible for 60 percent of one's weight and fat-bearing capacity in adulthood. The other 40 percent results from lifestyle and environmental cues interacting with genes. Genes are powerful, and so are our lifestyle choices and habits.

Energy Imbalance

Calories matter whether you choose to count or ignore them. The fundamental matter confronting personal nutrition is how many calories one's body can rightfully be entitled to in order to satisfy energy and nutrient needs. Excess calories beyond this requirement are handled by the body in two ways: greater calorie expenditure through activity or fat storage. No one, not even Americans, are exempt from the inexorable principle of calorie consumption balancing with calorie expenditure, better known as the *energy balance equation*.

The energy balance equation formulates the necessary conditions whereby weight is maintained, lost or gained. Energy intake must equal energy output to balance or maintain weight. When energy intake exceeds energy output, weight is gained. When energy output exceeds energy intake, weight is lost. All diets, despite their names, approaches and formulas, are necessarily based on the principle of energy balance whether or not they admit it, and whether or not they count calories or grams. Restriction of food and addition of physical activity are the only factors that we can consciously manipulate to effect negative balance of energy calories to lose weight.

If you are overweight or obese, you have a prolonged history of creating excess by consuming more than you are expending. The body has only two choices in managing excess: burning excess or storing excess. Any macronutrient in excess (whether fat, carbohydrates, or protein) can ultimately be converted to stored sugar or stored fat. The evolutionary role of fat is self-regulation. Taking cues from lifestyle and environment, the body knows when to burn off excess or store it for impending winter, non-fruiting season, famine, or pregnancy. Excess fat, in evolutionary terms, rendered an individual unattractive for sexual competition, burdensome to the rest of the pack, and a drain on precious natural resources better intended for fitter specimens to perpetuate the species.

If you are twenty pounds overweight, for example, you have 70,000 thousand calories in storage. Let's do the math together for those finding themselves thirty, forty, and fifty pounds overweight.

- 30 lbs x 3,500 calories per lb = 105,000 stored calories
- 40 lbs x 3,500 calories per lb = 140,000 stored calories

These are calories stored up for winter, famine, non-fruiting season, or pregnancy that never arrives. This is a lot of fat equity. Too bad these stored calories can't be redeemed for cash. That was the bad news. The good news is that every individual's God-given right to be thin is implied on both sides of the energy balance equation either as energy intake or energy output.

- Energy Intake = food consumed can be increased or reduced according to one's level of physical activity from sedentary to highly active.
- Energy Output = expenditure of calories can be increased according to four types of activity

Energy Output = Resting Metabolism + Thermic Effect of Food + Thermic Effect of Exercise + Non-Exercise Activity Thermogenesis (NEAT)

N.B. thermic or thermogenesis = calorie burning or heat generating

Small increments of calorie burning in each of these aspects of energy expenditure can effect fat reduction over a prolonged period of time, ASSUMING THAT NO NEW FAT HAS ACCUMULATED. Thus, a meaningful protocol for permanent fat loss must necessarily include two components: reduction of current fat stores and avoidance of new generations of fat stores.

Calorie energy fuels four types of metabolic activity:

- Basal or resting metabolic rate (BMR) (RMR) refers to calorie expenditure necessary to support bodily functions such as digestion, energy creation, cellular repair and regeneration, hormonal support, cardiac output, muscle contraction, brain control center, maintenance of organ and nervous systems, elimination and detoxification, and so forth. Since BMR/ RMR utilizes approximately 60 percent of total daily calorie expenditure, it offers the greatest opportunity for increased calorie burning primarily through development of muscle. One pound of added muscle, for example, burns 50 additional calories per day. Ten pounds of added muscle (a reasonable and laudable goal to strive for) burns 500 additional calories per day. Two important points to bear in mind: 1) the majority of daily calories are expended in just keeping us alive; 2) muscularity, not excess fat, drives metabolism.
- Thermic effect of food (TEF). The work of food digestion, appropriation, and assimilation of nutrients creates heat and raises metabolic rate as much as 10 to 15 percent of total daily calorie expenditure. Of the three macronutrients, protein produces the greatest thermic effect.
- Thermic effect of exercise (TEE) burns calories through working out and informal physical activity such as dancing, hobbies, gardening, and playing instruments. TEE utilizes 10 to 15 percent of total daily calorie expenditure.
- Non-exercise activity thermogenesis (NEAT) is a catch-all category of calorie burning that includes environmental/lifestyle components that do not neatly fit into previous categories such

as climate [exposure to cold], sickness, dietary overfeeding and dieting, and spontaneous or non-purposeful movement such as chores, fidgeting, gum chewing, surfing the Internet, sitting, and standing. NEAT utilizes 10 to 15 percent of total daily calorie expenditure.

Primal Solutions

Raising BMR/RMR offers the greatest opportunity for increased calorie burning because it involves a greater percentage of total daily calories. Small gains in lean muscle growth reap a higher yield in calorie expenditure since BMR/RMR accounts for 60 percent of total calories. Each component of the "energy output" side of the equation, however, gives us opportunity to burn more calories by:

- exercising to increase lean body mass, improve hormonal sensitivity, speed up metabolism, and stimulate new muscle growth
- increasing consumption of foods with good thermic effect (protein, raw plant foods, omega-3 and-6, fiber, and cold water and foods)
- staying physically active at home and at work with NEAT activity.

Chronic Dieting

All of us veteran dieters have learned that habitual dieting only guarantees two things: quick reduction of a few pounds (usually lean tissue and water not fat) and even quicker regaining of the same pounds plus more. Chronic dieting recycles the same old fat disguised in newer generations of fat. In addition to making us tired and cranky, dieting leaves us always dreaming of our next meal or snack. Satiety is constantly thwarted. The truly dark side of habitual dieting is its ability to activate famine mode in our genes or activate drought mode (the harbinger preceding famine) due to loss of body water. Episodic dieting achieves the opposite of its intention by slowing metabolism.

Primal Solution

Maintaining or speeding metabolism is the primary means of fat mobilization, not dieting which generally slows it down.

Content of Your Calories

All diets are guises for fastidious rationing of one, two, or all three macronutrients: low-carb, high-carb, low-fat, high-fat, low-protein, high-protein, and combinations of these. When one macronutrient increases, of course, another one necessarily decreases, unless all three of them more or less approach equality, as some diets propose. This quibbling of content is meaningful because nutritional content of meals and snacks is as important as calorie value. By making good eating choices, we obtain the full value of our calories for energy fuel as well as micronutrients that maximize health, longevity, and fat loss acceleration.

Good food choices promote easy digestion and absorption of nutrients. Having all three macronutrients (protein, fat and carbohydrate) present at meal and snack times balances blood sugar regulation and registers higher degree of satiety because fats and carbs release energy more easily than protein, which requires more calorie energy for digestion and metabolism yet satisfies longer.

Carbohydrates, both simple and complex (starches), have recently received the most criticism for creating epidemic proportions of obesity in the United States and globally. There is absolutely nothing inherently "bad" or "wrong" with carbs, but that our diets make exaggerated use of them. Consumption of all food types produces insulin hormone and especially excess carbohydrates that are refined and simple sugars. Overproduction of insulin eventually causes insulin resistance at cell receptor sites which inhibits blood sugar (glucose) regulation. Excess, rampant glucose is converted to glycogen for storage in the liver and muscles or to fat for storage in fat cells.

Primal Solutions

- Avoid or banish the most damaging carbohydrates, namely pure fruit juices (=liquid sugar), refined sugars (especially high-fructose corn syrup, sodas, and artificial, artificial/ chemical sweeteners), refined grains, and products that contain both refined sugars and refined grains such as sweetened/ flavored yogurts, breakfast cereals, breads, pastries, junk foods, and processed foods, energy drinks and candy.

- Don't be too fanatical about banning refined sugars and grains. You'll survive small doses of them here and there. Eventually, your taste buds will lose interest in pursuing excessive sweetness. Discover the sweet in everything you eat. You will find to your surprise that chewing almost any type of food long enough eventually produces a sweet taste. Don't swallow until you the find the "sweet" in every bite.

- For overall health and fat loss acceleration, restrict carbohydrate consumption to fiber-rich, enzyme-laden, nutrient-dense vegetables, nuts and seeds, whole fruits, whole grains, legumes, beans, fermented dairy products, and resistant starches.

- Get your five to nine daily servings of fruits and especially vegetables. Vegetables are like classical music. Our body and brain cells instinctively respond to them with ecstasy, but on the conscious level, we still have to work a little at enjoying them.

N.B. The etymological root of the word vegetable is Latin "vegetus" and "vegetare," meaning "life" and "to animate."

Nutrient Density (versus Designer Coffees, Juices, Energy Drinks, and 6-pk Mini Donuts)

Foods that are generally dense in nutrients are also sparse in calories, two exemplary qualities to have if you are a food. Essential and accessory nutrients such as fiber, enzymes, antioxidants, probiotics, plant compounds, vitamins, and minerals are extremely beneficial for promoting superior health. The body requires thousands of these nutrients in microscopic quantities to create vitality, the meaning of the word "vitamin." Micronutrients perform extraordinary tasks of cellular and DNA protection and regeneration, control free radical damage, aid in digestion and elimination, and assist in metabolic functions. The body does not store many micronutrients. On a daily basis, they need to be replaced as they are lost in respiration, perspiration, and elimination. (However, fat-soluble vitamins A, D, E and K can be stored in tissue.)

Many Americans are extremely deficient in micronutrients, especially minerals and trace elements. The most important meal to replenish micronutrients is breakfast. But not any old breakfast will do. A breakfast of mini donuts and black coffee, for example, might contain 360 calories, most of which is fat and sugar and extremely lacking in nutrients. The same number of calories could be exchanged for more wholesome and delicious fare such as the following example.

Whey protein shake + almond milk + raw egg + bowl of berries + banana (midmorning snack)		
Versus	=	*360 calories*
Six mini donuts + black coffee		

Primal Solution

Designer coffee drinks, caffeinated energy drinks, and fruit juices contain a similar number of calories and equally impoverished nutrition as the mini donut breakfast (above). Indulge in these only occasionally (if at all) and save some money, time, and your waistline.

Nutritional Deficiency

Sunlight, air, water, soil, bacteria, and food provide all the essential and accessory nutrients that magnify health and vitality in the human body. From these sources, we obtain oxygen, essential amino acids, essential fatty acids, vitamins, minerals, digestive aids (enzymes, probiotics, and friendly bacteria), herbs, and thousands of other micronutrients such as proteins, antioxidants, and plant chemicals.

The USDA asserts that typical American diets are woefully deficient in recommended daily INTAKE of "right" foods and grossly excessive in recommended daily LIMIT of "wrong" foods. We are walking around overfed yet undernourished. Our diets are seriously lacking in essential and accessory nutrients. Unhealthy eating patterns of Americans are sharply depicted in the following chart. Americans typically manage to obtain the following percentages of recommended daily/weekly intake of critical food substances.

Vegetables	59%	Fiber	40%
Fruits	42%	Potassium	56%
Seafood	44%	Vitamin D	28%
Dairy	52%	Calcium	75%
Whole Grains	15%	Oils	61%

On the other hand, typical American diets exceed their limits of recommended dietary intake of foods that should be minimized, as indicated below. The following foods should be used sparingly, mostly to enhance the palatability of nutrient-dense foods such as vegetables, whole grains, and proteins because Americans consume them in excess:

- solid fats and added sugars exceed the recommended limit by 180 percent.
- refined grains exceed the limit by 100 percent.
- sodium exceeds the limit by 49 percent.
- saturated fats exceed the limit by 10 percent.

Primal Solutions

Content as much as quantity of calories matters. According to this USDA data, Americans need to increase daily/weekly intake of vegetables, fruits, seafood, dairy products, whole grains, oils, fiber, potassium, calcium, and vitamin D. On the other hand, we need to limit daily/weekly intake of solid and saturated fats, added sugars, refined grains, and sodium. Not surprisingly, Americans tend to get adequate protein whether they are vegetarians or omnivores.

Diminished Diversity of Foods (Three Grains and Sugar Cane)

Your gut is an internal ecosystem that benefits from micro-biodiversity as much as large-scale ecosystems. For millions of years, our earliest ancestors hunted meat and gathered edible plant foods from a genetically diverse cornucopia of natural foods ranging from 10,000 to 50,000. Prehistoric humans gathered between 1,500 and

3,000 plant foods. On average, early humans ate some 800 varieties of plant foods. During the agricultural and industrial revolutions, human diets regularly consisted of 150 to 200 foods. Today, approximately 30 plants make up 95 percent of modern human nutrition. Of these, 9 are the source for 75 percent of carbohydrate energy in modern diets: wheat, corn, rice, barley, sorghum, potatoes, yams (sweet potatoes), sugar cane, and soy.

Industrial agriculture has further reduced our processed food diets to three grains and sugar cane: wheat, corn, and rice. These grains comprise 60 percent of total calories and protein calories that humans obtain from plants. Rice furnishes calories and protein for almost half of the world's population.

Whereas primal ancestors' diet consisted of extraordinary genetic diversity of plant foods plus meat and fish, modern diets, on the other hand, focus on animal flesh foods and limited menu of plant foods, for example, mostly fruits and vegetables. Over the course of human evolution, our diets have diminished exponentially in genetic diversity, giving way to wide variety of highly industrialized, mass-produced, concentrated foods manufactured from "three grains and sugar cane." The most nutritious elements of these grains, the germ and endosperm, have been stripped away and added back as synthetic nutrients. From adulterated, nutrient-deprived grains, we derive the following dietary staples, to mention a few: refined grains, refined sugars, artificial sweeteners, high-fructose corn syrup, boxed cereals, junk snack foods, caffeinated soft drinks, fruit concentrates, and juices.

In addition to diminished diversity of plant foods, American soil is diminished in quality to the point that the majority of Americans are seriously deficient in one or more micronutrients.

Primal Solution

Discover a new plant food every week at a local farmer's market, supermarket or organic garden.

Chromium Deficiency

Chromium is an essential micro-mineral that human (and animal) bodies require for regulating carbohydrate metabolism. This mineral enhances the effect of insulin for proper use of glucose (blood sugar). Deficiency of chromium therefore undermines blood sugar stability. Chromium is stored in many parts of the body, including muscles and fat as well as the skin, brain, spleen, kidneys, and testes. Known as the "ultra trace mineral" because the body needs only extremely tiny amounts to perform its essential functions, chromium is easy to be deficient in due to low absorption and high excretion rates in humans. The United States is known for its high incidence of chromium deficiency because of low soil levels of the mineral and overconsumption of refined foods such as sugar and sugar products, refined white flour, sodas, candies, breakfast cereals, white bread, and crackers. Better soil quality and less refined diets would significantly reverse the deficiency.

Primal Solutions

Good dietary sources of chromium include the following: brewer's yeast (stellar source of chromium), beef, liver, whole wheat, rye, fresh chilies, wheat germ and bran, oysters, onions, potatoes (especially the skins), tomatoes, green peppers, eggs, chicken, apple, butter, bananas, spinach, black pepper, molasses, whole grains, meats, shellfish, and many vegetables.

N.B. Two tablespoons of brewer's yeast provides 186 mcg or 155% of daily value for chromium.

Get the BAT to Beat Fat!

Ah, dear BAT! Where are you (at)?

The color of your fat makes a big difference in what happens to excess fat. Beautiful brown fat tissue located in discrete locations throughout the body symbolizes everybody's God-given right to be lean. Brown adipose fat (BAT) is the body's organ of caloric waste whereas white adipose fat tissue (WAT) is the body's organ of caloric storage. BAT is considered healthy, youthful fat while WAT is considered ugly, unhealthy visceral fat. BAT plays a fundamental role in fat management. It prevents fats consumed at meals from being stored as fat by burning it off (heat dissipation), plus it burns up stored calories acquired from stored WAT fat. Alas, BAT is abundant in our infancy and childhood but decreases significantly as we get older. Younger people have more BAT than older people. Lean people have more BAT than fat people. This is why we were able to eat seemingly whatever we wanted in our days of youth with impunity. Efficiency or dormancy of BAT is key to each person's fat profile. As little as 10 percent deficiency of BAT function can theoretically result in three or four dozen pounds of fat accumulation over the course of a normal lifetime. BAT is generally sluggish in most adult humans and it is difficult to compensate for the impact of this deficiency on health by dieting and exercising. The older you are, the more difficult it is to manage fat via BAT.

Primal Solutions

Wherever BAT resides or is activated, there is serious fat burning. Thermogenic (i.e. heat generating) substances and activities increase BAT fat management. When BAT activity increases, proper fat/lean body mass ratio improves. Thermogenics that assist in restoring BAT activity include the following:

- vigorous resistance training
- green tea extracts, ginger, licorice root, and cayenne pepper
- selected herbs, spices and roots like ma huang, yerba mate, kola nut, and guarana
- sea vegetables like kelp and bladderwrack
- protein consumption
- dietary nutrients of plant foods
- minerals like chromium, selenium, zinc, magnesium, potassium, and calcium
- vitamins C, B, and E
- essential fatty acids EFAs (the omegas) such as evening primrose, borage, flax, and black currant
- extended exposure to extreme temperatures, hot and cold (for example, drinking ice-cold water, taking cold showers, relaxing in saunas/hot tubs and vacationing in tropical climates)

N.B. Recent research on exercise and fitness suggests that resistance (anaerobic) training but not aerobic training triggers higher resting metabolic rate (RMR) and sustained fat burning many hours after intense exercise by means of a bonus effect known as excess post-oxygen consumption (EPOC).

Not Giving a Fat Rat: Negativity or Indifference

On top of multiple physiological causes, we often remain fat due to psychological reasons. After years of trial-and-error dieting, thwarted expectations and abandoned hope, it is difficult to overcome the inertia of negative thinking characterized by indecision, ambivalence, impatience, disgust, depression and "why me" syndrome. Yielding not to temptation while confronted on every hand by obesity-supportive marketing requires Victorian virtue. Feeling that you have put so much effort into fat reduction for so little result weighs heavily on the heart. Still we secretly harbor the hope that, because we are such decent, loving, and hardworking humans who have made valiant attempts to redeem our fat for lean, our excess fat will magically disappear with minimally inconvenient intervention on our part like *deus ex machina* of classical Greek tragedy. Finally, the surfeit of diet information—good, bad, junk, and pseudo—produces paralyzing consternation about how to transform ourselves even if we wanted to.

Primal Solutions

- Instead of being overly positive or negative in attitude, just witness yourself throughout the day, noticing whatever you notice. Witnessing is the state of being that is concerned with neither doing nor undoing.
- Be decisive and push past procrastination. Once you have gained momentum with decent results, then maximize it.

Aging

While the mind keeps track of calendar days,
the body keeps track of cellular malaise.

132

Aging is normal, inescapable consequence of living. Humans experience the aging process in two profound ways: biological and chronological. Aging deteriorates health in several ways. Sleep becomes more interrupted and less restorative. Mechanical parts erode and wear out. Mature bodies are more subject to accidents, bruising, and frailty. Memory fades. Eyesight blurs. Energy levels can fluctuate dramatically. Sexual libido wanes. Graying, thinning, and balding occur. Muscles and fat sag. Spinal integrity of our youth is compromised. Posture stoops due to difficulty in resisting gravity. Drug use increases (prescription, recreational, and over-the-counter). The normal aging process becomes even more accelerated with excess fat with its risk factors for a host of deleterious medical conditions including heart disease, the number-one killer of Americans, especially in overweight men.

Aging is experienced most profoundly at the level of cells and genes, the architects and engineers of our existence. Energy consumption and production as well as all life-sustaining mechanisms are negotiated in the mitochondria of our trillions of cells, including fat metabolism. Excess fat compromises normal cellular function. Excess fat stresses the body in myriad ways: cells are stressed due to rampant free radical damage, tissues become inflamed due to stress and toxic waste, hormones become imbalanced due to resistance at cell receptor sites, bodily fluids become acidic due to lack of alkaline foods and hydration, and organ systems falter due to energy imbalance and insufficient physical stimulation. All of these negative factors directly influence fat gain.

Aging and excess fat are two conditions that share commonalities. The same symptoms that characterize aging are the same symptoms that accelerate fat accumulation. By addressing either of these symptoms, the twin promises of anti-aging and lean body composition appear simultaneously obtainable. In other words, the same effort that successfully retards or reverses one condition will automatically do the same for the other with no extra effort.

Primal Solutions

Characterized below are conditions and solutions that contribute to aging and excess fat. Solutions are simple but not easy. Many threatening conditions of aging and excess fat gain can be ameliorated simply by adopting a healthy lifestyle that incorporates adequate sleep, regular exercise, and managed stress along with a balanced diet replete in plant-rich whole foods.

Conditions	Solutions
Loss of lean muscle	High-intensity interval training and cardio workouts
Loss of bone mass	Weight-bearing exercise and mineral nutrition
Loss of lung capacity	Short, intense cardiopulmonary exercise
Increased fat storing	Hormonal sensitivity of insulin and leptin
Decreased fat burning	Activation of brown adipose fat BAT
Dormant human growth hormone	Sleep and regular exercise (moderate to intense)
Inactive fast-twitch muscle fibers	Frequent, short, intense exercise
Low lean-to-fat body ratio	Muscle-building and fat-burning
Nutritional deficiency	Varied and nutrient-dense diet, probiotics, and enzymes
Cellular damage	Antioxidants to bombard free radicals
Telomere shortening in DNA	Anti-aging, longevity practices
Hormonal resistance	Regulation of blood sugar levels along with balanced diet
Sleep deprivation	Melatonin sensitivity and minimal rampant cortisol

Free Radical Damage or Oxidative Stress

Oxidative stress or free radical damage in cells is the root cause of many disorders. It occurs when undetached (free), unstable oxygen and nitrogen-containing molecules steal ions from stable molecules. If antioxidants do not overpower free radicals, damage to protein, fat, and DNA cells ensues. Although free radicals play a positive role in immune function as they defend us against rogue bacteria and viruses, we generally despise them for their thuggish behavior prevailing in the decent neighborhoods of our cells and genes. Free radicals are unstable, unpaired oxygen molecules (reactive oxygen species or ROS) that steal from other paired molecules to stabilize themselves. They cause oxidative stress to our cells and genes by altering, damaging, and destroying cell membranes and the genetic code of DNA. Oxygen is indispensable to all that lives and breathes even to free radicals. Paradoxically, breathing is the activity that produces the greatest amount of free radicals. Fats are highly unstable chemical substances that contain oxygen. Oxidized fatty acids become primary fuel for certain cancers in various organs.

Runaway free radical damage causes our cells to rust, age, mutate, and degenerate. As cells degenerate, so do organ systems. As we age, our natural ability to control free radical damage significantly declines, requiring enormous nutritional support of antioxidants. The longer we live and breathe, the more free radicals we create. Truly, to breathe is to age. Alas, you cannot avert the problem by holding your breath.

Primal Solutions

The plant kingdom reigns supreme in aiding us to combat free radical damage with exponential numbers of powerful antioxidants and health-supportive nutrients. But the most powerful antioxidants reside internal to our very own body and can be found in every one of our trillions cells. Their names are glutathione and alpha-lipoic acid.

To combat oxidative stress of free radicals, it is important to fortify ourselves with nutritional support of essential nutrients and plant compounds of which only about 4,000 out of many thousands are currently identified.

- Drink teas high in antioxidants (green, red, white, and black).
- Eat nutrient-rich plant and animal foods that supply Omega-3 fatty acids (ALA, EPA, and DHA), fat-soluble vitamins (A, D, E, and K and beta-carotene), water-soluble vitamins (C), B-complex vitamins, and selenium (mineral).
- Emphasize foods rich in antioxidant protection including fats and oils, spices, herbs, fruits, and vegetables (the darker in color, the richer in plant compounds), red wine, dark chocolate, teas, and coffee.
- Boost the body's own master antioxidants, glutathione and alpha-lipoic acid, with foods that enhance their production.

Glutathione is the body's master antioxidant. Scientists speculate that glutathione was essential to the very development of life on the earth because no living organisms, plants or animals, exist without it. Glutathione is made naturally in every cell. Maintaining high levels of glutathione is critical to life for reasons such as removing toxins from cells, protecting DNA from oxidative stress caused by free radicals, maintaining healthy liver function, reducing chronic inflammation, boosting immune function, promoting structural integrity of red blood cells, detoxifying pollutants and carcinogens, and neutralizing radiation. In addition, glutathione is a neurotransmitter. As we age, the body's ability to produce glutathione diminishes.

Excellent food choices that enhance glutathione production are mostly fruits and vegetables, preferably consumed raw or lightly cooked. These foods are asparagus, avocados, potatoes, spinach, okra, strawberries, white grapefruit, peaches, oranges, cantaloupe, watermelon, dark green, leafy vegetables, broccoli, cabbages, tomatoes, wheat germ, oats, ricotta and cottage cheeses, and walnuts. All meats are high in amino acid cysteine, one of the building blocks of glutathione.

Alpha-lipoic acid is the body's super-antioxidant. It is revered for the ability to defend every type of substance against oxidative assaults on both fluids (like blood) and fatty tissues (like cell membranes). Alpha-lipoic acid is amazing for its water and fat solubility. Further, it guards against strokes, heart attacks, and cataracts, strengthens memory, turns off genes that express aging and cancer, and helps the body break down sugar for energy production. Like glutathione, alpha-lipoic acid is synthesized right in the body itself from amino acids. Foods like spinach, broccoli, Brussels sprouts, tomatoes, potatoes, and peas deliver small amounts of alpha-lipoic acid. One can boost levels of alpha-lipoic acid with the following supplements that are well documented and safe: Coenzyme Q10, Acetyl-L-carnitine (ALCAR), N-acetylcysteine (NAC), berry extracts with anthocyanins, lutein, and green tea and green tea extracts.

- Address stress in your life through awareness, sleep, rest, relaxation and meditation techniques, yoga, free play, spontaneous activities, sports, hobbies, creativity, and volunteerism.

Inflammation

Fat cells secrete all kinds of inflammatory compounds so overweight people are very likely to have high levels of inflammation. Most of us are aware that inflammation is linked to heart disease and a host of other scary conditions. Many medical researchers believe that excess inflammation is the root cause of most diseases. Inflammation plays a critical role in the body's self-defense mechanism that keeps us healthy. It is a normal condition of the body that has to be balanced by pro-inflammatory and anti-inflammatory substances. Omega-6 foods evoke pro-inflammatory responses in the body whereas omega-3 foods evoke anti-inflammatory responses. Oxidation (metabolism) of arachidonic acid, a highly unsaturated and unstable fatty acid derived from the omega-6 parent linoleic acid, serves as the primary fuel for cancer growth in various organs.

Primal Solutions

The best strategy for controlling the fires of inflammation is three-pronged:

- Prevent additional inflammation from occurring by cutting down but not eliminating omega-6 foods prominent in your diet. (A penny of prevention is worth a pound of cure.)
- Increase omega-3 foods in the diet without becoming excessive or obsessive.
- Strike a balance between omega-3 and-6 foods that approaches the ideal of our pre-agricultural past of 1:1 to 1:4. Most American diets have ratios as high as 1 (omega-3) to 25 (omega-6).

Moderate Omega-6 foods in your diet including fats and oils extracted from seeds and grains, for example, cottonseed, corn, safflower, sunflower, soybean, fish high in omega-6, and grain-based processed foods (cereals, pastries, and snack foods). Omega-3 foods such as the following extinguish the fires of inflammation: seeds and oils from flax, chia (salba), perilla, walnut, medicinal herbs, spices, and fish and coldwater fatty fish such as salmon, sardines, trout, herring, mackerel, and anchovies.

Medicinal herbs and spices have been revered for thousands of years in cultures worldwide for their significant inhibitory effects on inflammation and pain relief. Among the most majestic substances are ginger, turmeric, green tea, holy basil, oregano, rosemary, feverfew, hops, Baikal skullcap, Chinese goldthread, barberry, and Hu-zhang (Japanese knotweed). Ginger alone contains 477 constituents, including multiple enzymes and melatonin that work synergistically with inherent ingredients. Combining multiple herbs produces profoundly beneficial effects on human physiology.

Mild to moderate exercise and meditation are known to lower levels of inflammation. Any success in lowering inflammation levels also lowers one's risk for multiple conditions for which inflammation is the underlying (and unsuspected) cause.

Acidity

Human bodies contain 70 percent water and fluids. Blood is 90 percent water. Excess acidity of blood and body fluids is responsible for a host of symptoms and illnesses. Excess acidity contributes to weight gain because the body compensates (buffers the acidity) by leaching precious alkaline minerals such as calcium, potassium, magnesium, and sodium from bone mass and lean muscle tissue to restore acid-base balance to fluids. More important for fat loss, the body makes fat and cholesterol to neutralize acids in the blood and body tissues as defense mechanism to pack away the acids to keep them from eroding vital organs.

Diets high in protein content increase acidity. Even mildly acidic environments in body fluids lead to loss of bone mineral. Loss of bone mineral and loss of lean muscle are co-conspirators in weight gain.

Oxygen levels drop in acidic environments, creating ideal conditions for pathogens (bacteria, viruses, and fungus) to thrive. Alkaline foods neutralize acidity, ameliorating overly acidic internal environment and giving the body less reason to maintain or create fat.

Primal Solutions

Rather than reaching for Tums or Milk of Magnesia, take a major step in reducing highly acidic environments of your body fluids by reducing dietary intake of acidic foods and beverages and increasing alkaline foods and beverages. Avoid overconsumption of meats, sweets, grains, legumes, dairy products, and starches like breads and pastries. Organic vegetables are primary sources of highly alkaline minerals. They should be included in every meal. Emphasize foods listed below because they are alkaline or highly alkaline foods.

Vegetables	All vegetables especially green ones, potatoes, and sweet potatoes
Salad greens	Lettuces, dandelion, chicory, escarole, and arugula
Green vegetables	Spinach, cooking greens (e.g. kale, collards, mustards, turnips)beet greens, green cabbage, artichoke, Brussels sprouts, and celery
Other vegetables	Carrots, fennel, red cabbage, and yellow beans
Fruiting vegetables	Tomatoes, cucumber, sweet peppers, zucchini, squash, and edible gourds
Green herbs	Parsley, basil, rosemary, peppermint, and cilantro
Fruits	Berries, bananas, and citrus fruits
Nuts	Almonds, Brazil nuts, almond milk, and soymilk
Grains	Corn

Dairy	Raw whole milk, whole pasteurized milk, fresh butter, fresh whey, fresh buttermilk, and egg yolks *Exclude whole milk if it is homogenized, sterilized, or ultra-pasteurized*
Condiments	Sea salt, table salt, raw cane sugar (Sucanat), pear concentrate, blackstrap molasses, and apple cider vinegar
Liquids	Pure water, mineral water, alkalized water with pH of 7.4 or higher, coconut water, and herbal teas
Fats	Extra-virgin olive oil (cold-pressed), safflower oil, sunflower oil, and fresh butter

X

Getting Started Now!

Planning, Patience, and High Resolve = Victory

Resolve psychological ambivalence about your fat loss efforts by staying committed to a viable strategic plan no matter what! Fat is gained and lost by imperceptible increments. Being in a hurry to reverse years, decades, and perhaps even a whole lifetime of fat gain will surely undermine the most valiant efforts. Grant yourself a year or two, which is little time in comparison to years and decades it took you to get to your present condition. The body is miraculous. It actually wants to be what you are striving for it to become. Apply some *Horse-Sense Nutrition* and see how magically the body uncovers its true lean self.

By now you should be convinced that a multiple-prong approach to fat loss is the most effective. Let's call this our triple-B's strategy:

- boost metabolism
- build muscle
- burn fat

Nutrition is the common denominator for employing this strategy. Central to optimal nutrition is the inclusion of plant foods that, above all benefits, create a hospitable environment for digestive wellness which is the foundation for maximizing metabolism, increasing muscle mass, and burning fat more efficiently. You have also become convinced by now that in nutrition terms you only need to make minor shifts with regard to proteins and fats and a major shift with regard to carbohydrates. Let's call this strategy: paradigm shifts regarding fork lifts.

Proteins. Whether omnivore or vegetarian, most Americans get sufficient protein. Our goal regarding this macronutrient concerns two things: to procure cleaner, higher quality sources of protein, namely, organic, pasture-fed meats; and to consume more plant sources of protein especially green leafy vegetables.

Fats. Most American bodies could stand an oil change. This change relates to three aspects: to obtain more omega 3-6-9 fats primarily from nuts and seeds in balanced ratio; to use saturated fats and oil in moderation for cooking, frying, and baking; and to use unsaturated fats and oils for non-cooking purposes.

Carbohydrates. The foods that are implicated for contributing the most to the global obesity epidemic are manufactured foods made primarily with white flour and white sugar combined with high fat in thousands of products. These foods are absolutely dispensable, useless calories. The plant kingdom supplies all our nutritive needs through fruits, vegetables, flowers, stems, leaves, roots, legumes, mushrooms, nuts, seeds and whole grains gathered from land, sea, forest, field and desert. The glory of the plants foods is that they supply a vast array of diverse micronutrients which cost practically zero calories. Many of them can be eaten in nearly unlimited quantity.

The Magic Bullet of Fat Loss: Plant Foods (Roots, Stems, Leaves, Flowers, Seeds, Nuts, and Fruits)

Humans and green plants share a deep chemical bond. You could say that we are even blood-related. Plant chlorophyll and human blood have the same chemistry except for one molecular difference, magnesium in chlorophyll and iron molecules in human blood. All nutritive material that we derive from animal flesh originally came from plants, soil, sunlight, and water.

Plants are the most numerous species on our planet, and we, animals and humans alike, are needy dependents of their goodness and bounty. If there ever were a happy ending to the story of our banishment from the Garden of Eden, it is this. Despite the woes that perpetually plague us in every arena of modern life, we remain ever surrounded by the essence of garden plant life: fruits, vegetables, roots, stems, leaves, flowers, seeds, nuts, legumes, grasses, saps, barks, mushrooms, and sea plants. Plant foods are our nutritional superstars and saviours. They fill us and heal us. As long as we were able to find a leaf or root, we humans could survive. The plant kingdom was indispensable to our survival as a species and continues to play a stellar role in helping us thrive today. When we eat plant foods, primal knowledge encoded in our cells interacts with intelligence locked up in plant cells. This interaction of human and plant cells harmonizes and balances our inner ecology. The curative power of plant foods cleanses, detoxifies, heals, and keeps our figures attractive and fit. To address the root cause of excess fat or any health condition, we need only to eat more roots. Roots are plant foods, not foods from manufactured plants. They are delicious multi-vitamin/ mineral pills that, despite the exquisite beauty and virtuous sensuality, we hesitate to swallow because they don't seem to go down the gullet as seductively as refined carbs and sugars.

Vegetables and fruits are the best source of natural sugars along with many other essential and accessory nutrients, thousands of which remain unidentified. Plant foods are our best allies because they help us fight for our overall health in general and fat loss in particular.

The unglamorous magic bullet of fat loss is eating more plant foods for their volume, satiety, chemical compounds, calorie sparsity, fiber, alkalinity, and antioxidant protection. Adhering to your plan of daily intake of five to nine plant food servings will do wonders for every aspect of your being. This substantial intake assists fat loss in the following ways:

- crowds out unneeded calories.
- satisfies energy and nutritional needs, the true basis of hunger and satiety.
- assuages our sweet tooth with natural sugars.

Follow the easy-to-execute plan on the next few pages. This action is the foundation of your physical transformation.

Your Planner of 5 to 9 Plant Foods Daily/Weekly Intake

Save Tons of Money and Plan Meals on a Weekly Basis

This plan is not about carb denial or restriction but addition and liberation. Vegetables and fruits are premium nutrition. Many people achieve impressive fat loss results simply by changing the content of their calories, replacing useless, calorie-dense foods calories with the full spectrum of rainbow-colored fruits and vegetables. For the price of a designer coffee/tea, energy drink, or pure fruit juice, you could be enjoying two to four servings of organic fruits or vegetables that infuse your physical being with calories and content that matter.

Goal: I will enjoy five to nine plant food servings per day within five weeks.

Vegetables and fruits are nutritional superstars and custodians of fat loss. Plan your meals and snacks around them, including raw, sun-ripened, biogenic (live and life-giving), photogenic vegetables and fruits, whole and juiced. The primary role of live plant foods is to cleanse and detoxify the body and supply nutrients, for example, fiber, enzymes, vitamins, minerals, amino acids, antioxidants, anti-inflammatories, phytochemicals, and chlorophyll.

Week 1

Start with five servings (=1/2 to 1 cup), for example:

1. lemon juice (freshly squeezed) with water (warm or room temperature) in the early morning for cleansing and detoxification
2. melons (cantaloupe or watermelon) prior to breakfast for more cleansing and detox
3. berries (fresh) as dessert or with whipped cream or with shortcake or with breakfast omelet
4. nuts or seeds or nut/seed milks (protein shakes) as a morning or afternoon snack
5. salad (huge volume) of dark, leafy greens with dinner

Week 2

Add a 6th serving, for example: legumes (soup beans or peas/lentils, chili con carne, hummus, or black bean salsa).

Week 3

Add a 7th serving, for example: resistant starch (potato salad, three-bean salad, cold vegetarian pasta dish, or sweet potato pie).

Week 4

Add an 8th serving, for example: whole grains (oats, rice, corn, quinoa, tabouli, popcorn snack, or rice pudding dessert).

Week 5

Add a 9th serving, for example: red wine (cabernet sauvignon, petite syrah, merlot) or grape juice

Now It's Time to Commit to Adequate Intake of Plant Foods

List five plant foods to incorporate into your daily nutrition for Week 1. A selected list of plant foods follows. Many other possibilities are available.

Suggested List of Plant Foods

For your five to nine daily servings, choose mostly from these categories of foods most of which are nutrient-dense and non-acid-producing. Emphasize berries, lemons, limes, greens (salad and cooking), green (cruciferous) vegetables, onion, garlic, mushrooms, nuts, and seeds.

Fruits

- berries
- citrus: lemons, limes, grapefruit, or oranges
- melons
- tropical: bananas, pineapple, or papaya

- sweet: apples, pears, grapes, mangos, cherries, peach, or nectarines
- fatty: avocados or olives
- others: tomatoes, pomegranates, persimmons, dates, or figs

Vegetables

- leafy greens (all)
- green: asparagus, celery, parsley, cucumber, peas, or green beans
- sprouts (all)
- sea vegetables (all)
- peppers: sweet and hot
- cruciferous: broccoli, cauliflower, cabbage, or Brussels sprouts
- allium: onion, garlic, or leeks
- root (tuber): carrots, beets, potatoes, yams, sweet potatoes, turnips, parsnips, gingerroot, or radishes
- gourds: squash or zucchini
- woods: mushrooms
- desert: aloe vera
- herbs, fresh and dried (all)
- spices

Legumes

- black beans
- kidney beans
- pinto beans
- white (navy) beans
- chick peas (garbanzo)
- lima bean
- black-eyed peas

- lentils
- granulated soy
- tofu
- soy flour
- soy nuts
- soy lecithin

Nuts/Seeds and Nut/Seed Butters

- almonds
- coconut
- flax seed
- macadamia
- sesame
- walnuts
- Brazil nuts
- chia seeds
- cumin seeds
- fennel seeds
- caraway seeds
- hempseed

Fats and Oils

- unsaturated: flaxseed, hempseed, black currant, olive, evening primrose, borage, and marine oils
- saturated: coconut

Grains/Grasses

- sprouted grains and grasses (all)

- amaranth
- buckwheat
- millet
- quinoa
- wild rice
- brown rice
- oats
- barley

Sweeteners

- stevia
- agave nectar
- blackstrap molasses
- coconut nectar

Condiments

- apple cider vinegar
- balsamic vinegar
- miso

Beverages

- water
- alkaline water
- distilled water
- teas (green, rooibos, white, yerba mate, fruit, or herbal)
- fresh coconut water
- red wine

My Five to Nine Daily Planner for Plant Foods Intake

Goal: Consuming these nourishing plant foods will help me achieve superior health and fitness and a uniquely (*You*-niquely) gorgeous body.*(Refer to the model from the previous pages.)*

Week 1

Start with five servings. (Most servings equal ½ to 1 cup.)

_____ a.m.

_____ a.m.

_____ a.m. or p.m.

_____ p.m.

_____ p.m.

Week 2

Add a 6th serving.

_____ a.m. or p.m.

Week 3

Add a 7th serving.

_____ a.m. or p.m.

Week 4

Add an 8th serving.

_____ a.m. or p.m.

Week 5

Add a 9ᵗʰ serving.

_____ a.m. or p.m.

Give yourself a grade (0 to 100 percent) as you complete each daily assignment of five to nine servings. Well done!

C.H.E.A.T with Superstar Fat Loss Accelerators and Members of High Satiety

Consider featuring the following foods prominently in your daily/ weekly planner of plant foods intake.

C = COCONUT

- Its high alkalinity (non-acidic) promotes release of stored toxins in fat tissue.
- It is loaded with minerals, especially magnesium and potassium (balanced with sodium), and low in calories.
- It has natural sugars. There is zero fat in coconut water and good fat in oil and cream. It has amino acids and vitamins.
- Its fat is medium-chain triglycerides excellent for fat burning and not fat storing like other saturated oils.
- It has similar chemical composition to human blood plasma and mother's milk.
- It has many forms/uses: water, oil, raw cream, flour, and curry.

H = HEMPSEED

- It is a raw protein source with complete spectrum of essential amino acids plus contains edestin (main protein of DNA cells) and albumin (main protein of human blood).
- It supplies perhaps the best ratio of omega-3 and-6 EFAs, plus it contains omega-9 and EPA, DHA, GLA, and SDA fatty acids important for production of hormones and prostaglandin. One tablespoon supplies RDI for omega-3.
- Its essential fatty acids are not energy fuel but are used for structural components of cell membranes, cardiovascular health, and inflammatory response. EFA deficiency is the prelude to many diseases.
- It has many forms/uses: seeds, oil, butter, raw protein powder, or meal.

E = EGGS

- They contain superior protein bioavailability score (94/100) and contains all essential amino acids.
- They are low calorie without carbohydrates. As germinative food, eggs contain all essential nutrients for sustaining life of its species.
- They contain biotin, choline, lutein, and cholesterol for forming brain cells.
- They have many forms/uses: omelets, quiches, egg salad, deviled, custards, and shakes.

A = AVOCADOS

- They have excellent protein and are fiber-rich. They are loaded with minerals, fat-burning enzymes, and lecithin.
- They have high satiety factor and are high in enzymes, including lipase for fat burning. They are packed with vitamins.
- They are great monounsaturated fats, which should contribute 70 percent of daily fat nutrition.
- They have many forms/uses: raw, guacamole, gazpacho, sandwich spread, salsa, and salad dressing.

T = TEA (green, unfermented) or Yerba Mate

- It is China's and South America's divine herb. It is high in antioxidants and inhibits cancers and tumors.
- Its caffeine has a thermic effect (heat creation/calorie burning) and raises metabolic rate.
- It has three healing properties: flavonoids, fluoride, and caffeine. It fights bacterial infections and improves mental clarity.
- It oxidizes fat and lowers blood lipids. It is alkalizing and anti-aging and does not contain calories or fat.
- It has many forms and uses: hot or cold beverage; sautéing vegetables.

XI

Imaginative Meal Planning:
Blessed Be the Tines That Bind

Meals are easier to eat than plan and implement. Balanced meal composition is critically important to insure that daily food intake will sufficiently supply appropriate raw materials for energy fuel and nutrients. Eating is recreational beyond fulfilling these two basic requirements.

Human and animal physiology are organized by internal mechanisms of hunger and appetite control for regulating when and how much to eat. The biological imperative of survival is met through eating. Hunger pangs register pain that is only alleviated by replenishment of energy fuel and nutrients. (Americans tend to emphasize need for fuel over need for nutrients.) The ultimate experience of pleasure is satiety registered collectively by the mouth, gut, and brain interacting with food and water. Primordial biological urges program us to live to eat as well as eat to live.

Satiety is the simplest and most comprehensive design principle of imaginative meal planning. Plan your meals around this concept. Eat them to the point of satiety and not a morsel more! Satiety is registered by the mouth, gut, and brain in a number of ways. Here are some:

SATIETY = control of hunger and appetite

SATIETY = response to volume, variety, and sensory stimulation

SATIETY = frequency of eating

SATIETY = synergy of protein, carbohydrates, and fat combined meals and snacks

SATIETY = reduction of blood sugar volatility

SATIETY = promotion of blood sugar stability

SATIETY = nutrient adequacy

SATIETY = calorie density

SATIETY = long duration of meals

SATIETY = communion with others during meals

SATIETY = fiber

SATIETY = water, vegetables juices, water-filled vegetables and fruits

SATIETY = large volumes of low-calorie nutritious plant foods

SATIETY = fat-enhanced proteins and carbohydrates

Proper Hydration: Drink, Drink, Drink

Dehydration compromises all metabolic systems, nutrient assimilation, elimination of toxins, and fat-burning processes. Hydrating your body responsibly aids cellular processes, energy expenditure and production, and fat burning. Ideal body composition cannot be attained without full hydration; muscle mass cannot be built without alkalized, oxygenated blood. We need water rehydration for the following reasons:

- Water constitutes 70 percent of the human body, 94 percent of human blood, 75 percent of muscles and heart, 83 percent of kidney and brains, 86 percent of lungs, 95 percent of eyes, and even 22 percent of seemingly dry bones. Each day, a substantial quantity of two quarts (eight cups), lost through perspiration, respiration, elimination, and metabolic functions, does not get adequately replaced.

- Researchers believe that 75 percent of Americans are chronically dehydrated, averaging about four glasses a day instead of the recommended seven to eight. An estimated 70 percent of Americans are going around chronically depleted.

* Caffeine drinks are diuretics, depleting the body of fluids along with precious minerals.
* Foods we eat are dried out, cooked to death, hard to swallow, and ingested too fast, requiring overtime work from saliva, enzymes, and gastric juices.

Precede each snack and meal with a glass of water. The greater the water content of your body composition, the less it consists of fat.

Snacks: Nutritious and Delicious

The purpose of snacks is three-pronged like a fork: to stave off hunger, keep blood sugar balanced, and supply calorie energy. Eat snacks only as needed. The following list enumerates delectable foods considered weight-loss weapons because they are packed with vitamins, minerals, amino acids, healthy fats, enzymes, fiber, antioxidants, distilled water, and other vital compounds. Life-producing foods such as fruits, nuts, and seeds are particularly great snack choices. The list includes: berries (fresh and dried), fruits (sweet, tropical, fatty, or dried), raw vegetables (crudités), hummus or salsa, green smoothies, coconut water, dairy products, eggs (hard-boiled or deviled), nuts and seeds, nut/seed butters, nut and grain milks, protein shakes, legumes (peanuts), large mixed salads, canned tuna, sardines, sea vegetables, homemade or canned soups, and teas (herbal, caffeinated, decaffeinated, or fruit). Avoid pure fruit juices because they are too sugary.

Meal Guidelines

- Strive to alkalize (the opposite of acidify) your meals by incorporating more raw or lightly cooked foods. A ratio of 60/40 raw to cooked foods is respectable.
- Design meals around an adequate portion of quality protein.
- Animal proteins are complete proteins. Dairy and eggs are protein foods. While some plant foods are complete proteins, others plant foods considered incomplete become complete proteins when combined throughout the day with other complementary plant foods.
- Supplement portions of protein with generous quantities of vegetables, water-filled, fibrous, low sugar, and non-starchy. Choose from dark, leafy greens, cooking greens, roots, bulbs, stems, flowers, mushrooms, sea vegetables, and edible weeds. Vegetables are the only category of foods that can be eaten in almost unlimited quantities. Large salads should be your daily vitamin. Eat vegetables uncooked and cooked.
- Add just enough fat to make the carbohydrates and proteins of your meal more palatable.
- Supplement with essential fatty acids omega-3 and-6 two or three times a week as whole foods or supplement form. Omega-3 foods include flax and chia seeds, walnuts, and wild caught coldwater, fatty fish. Omega-6 foods include nuts, seeds, grains, vegetable oils, and animal foods.
- Replace meals occasionally with protein shakes and green smoothies, for example, whey, soy, goat, egg, rice, and hemp protein. Green plant food smoothies are quality plant protein.
- Add small quantities of unrefined plant foods such as legumes and whole grains to meals.

- Substitute starches, especially resistant starches, for legumes and whole grains in meals.
- Tolerate recreational calories on special occasions. (See appendix for recipes.)
- In truth, all calories not intended or utilized for nutrition or calorie fuel purposes are recreational or discretionary calories. Discretionary calories as embodied in the recipes in the appendix can be tolerated on rare special occasions. Immediately afterward, get back on track with penitential care.

XII

RECIPES

Take Thyme to Become
a Salad Queen or King

One of the best habits you can develop to combat excess weight is grabbing a fork and eating a salad. Not the old tired salads with iceberg lettuce and Thousand Island dressing. I mean real ones fit for royalty. Yes, you. Salads should be routinely eaten on a daily basis. Few dishes offer such exemplary nutrient density and calorie sparsity. Salads serve equally well for breakfasts and snacks as for main meals. Although preparation of salads can admittedly be time-consuming, they also can be thrown together in minutes. Homemade dressings are easy and quick to whip up. You will save money and find yours far superior to commercial versions.

The concept of salads is simple: rinse, chop, mix, and eat. Innumerable recipes are available online or in superb books on salads like the following three: *Raising the Salad Bar* by Catherine Walthers; *Salad* by Williams-Sonoma; and *Salad* by *Cooking Light*. In addition to being delicious, salads are nutritionally virtuous in the following ways.

Unlimited Variety

Incorporate plants and animal foods (land and sea). Stimulate all the sensory organs: sight, smell, touch, taste, and hearing with their colors, shapes, textures, temperatures, tastes (sweet, sour, salty, bitter, and meaty or umami), and sounds (snap, crackle, and pop).

Fullness and Satisfaction

Salads can be eaten in almost unlimited quantity. Volume plus variety are high satiety factors for the mouth, gut and brain.

Cornucopia of Plant Foods

Choose from leafy greens, edible weeds, sprouts, herbs, spices, root and cruciferous vegetables, and fruits (citrus, fatty, spicy, sweet, and tropical).

Rainbow Colors

Design a decorative array of pigments with their attendant plant compounds: purple, red, blue, green, orange, yellow, and white.

Quality Proteins

Employ the full spectrum of essential and non-essential amino acids found in high-quality proteins.

Micronutrient Density

Incorporate a wide variety of plant foods which are natural powerhouses of vitamins, minerals, amino acids, fatty acids, antioxidants, fibers, enzymes, plant pigments, chlorophyll, distilled water, and anti-inflammatory agents.

Low Glycemic Load

Control blood sugar and insulin production with fibrous, low sugar vegetables, fruits, nuts, seeds, herbs, spices.

Elimination and Detoxification

Promote bowel evacuation and cleansing for intestinal health with a wide range of fibers, herbs, spices, roots, probiotics, and fermented foods.

List of Common Ingredients for Salads

Don't let the following list of ingredients overwhelm you. A salad can be made with just about anything. Use the opportunity to clean out your refrigerator while making salads. Forget the list and just be creative. Remember that green is the premium color for human and animal nutrition.

Greens	arugula, asparagus, beet greens (tops), bok choy, broccoli, broccoli rabe, cabbage, carrot tops, celery, chards, collard greens, dandelion, endive, escarole, frisée, iceberg lettuce, kale, mizuna, mustard greens, radish tops, red leaf lettuce, romaine lettuce, turnip greens, spinach, watercress
Edible Green Weeds (Wild Plants)	chickweed, cloves, dandelion greens and flowers, lamb's-quarter, malva, miner's lettuce, plantain, purslane, stinging nettles (parboiled)
Green Sprouts	alfalfa, broccoli, clover, fenugreek, radish, sunflower
Green Herbs	aloe vera, baby dill, basil, cilantro, fennel, mint, parsley, peppermint, spearmint, thyme
Raw Vegetables	beets (root), carrot (root), cabbage, celeriac, fennel, mushroom, radish (root), peppers (sweet and hot)
Roasted or Lightly Cooked Vegetables	asparagus, beet (root), peas, squash, sweet potato
Fruits	apple, asian pear, avocado, cucumber, olives, pear, raisins, tomato
Dried Berries	acai, goji
Seeds	chia (salba), flax, hempseed, pumpkin, sesame, squash, sunflower, wheat germ
Nuts	almond, beechnut, Brazil nut, cashew, pistachio, pecan, walnut
Sprouted Seeds, Legumes, and Grains	chickpea (garbanzo or ceci), lentils, rice, wild rice, quinoa, tabbouleh, couscous, pumpkin, sunflower, wheatgrass
Cooked Legumes	black-eyed pea, kidney, pinto, cannellini
Fats and Oils	almond, avocado, canola, coconut, hazelnut, olive, peanut, sesame, walnut, wheat germ
Vinegars	apple cider, balsamic, champagne, fig balsamic, red wine, rice
Condiments for Salad Dressings	anchovy fillets, bacon bits (not fake), capers, Dijon mustard, garlic, miso, pesto, raw egg yolk

Cooked Meats	wild tuna (canned), bacon bits (not fake), blackened catfish, farmed trout, mackerel, pancetta, smoked salmon, wild salmon, free-range chicken, hard-boiled egg, grass-fed beef, organic pork, shellfish (crab, lobster, scallops, shrimp)
Spices	black pepper (freshly ground), cayenne pepper, chili powder, cumin, ginger, sea salt, turmeric
Sea Vegetables	kelp, dulse, hijiki, arame
Juice, Peel, and Zests	grapefruit, lemon, orange
Cheeses	hard and soft; pasteurized and raw
Natural Sweeteners	agave nectar, coconut flesh, coconut nectar, coconut water, dates, honey, syrup, fruit juice
Miscellaneous	brewer's yeast, nutritional yeast

Enhance the experience of eating salads by serving them regally with your nicest dinner-and silverware. Now that you have become a salad queen/king, straighten up your crown. It's a little crooked.

Just Desserts

Eggcellent General Custard

Ingredients

- 1 cup heavy whipping cream and 1 cup single cream
- 1 cup milk
- 1 vanilla bean, split and seeds scraped into the cream/milk mixture. One teaspoon of vanilla extract can be substituted for the bean (the secret ingredient).
- 2 whole eggs plus 3 egg yolks
- 1/2 cup sugar (caster or superfine). Regular sugar suffices.

Preheat oven to 325 degrees.

Place cream, milk, vanilla bean (or extract), and seeds in a saucepan over medium to high heat until the mixture just comes to a boil. Do not overboil. Remove from heat and set aside. Combine eggs, extra yolks, and sugar in a bowl. Whisk until well combined.

Gradually add the hot cream mixture to the egg mixture, whisking well to combine. Pour into ramekins or a six-cup ovenproof pan.

Place water in long pan or deep-sided dish approximately half the height of the ramekins or ovenproof pan. Bake forty-five to fifty minutes or until done.

Remove the ramekins or ovenproof dish from the water bath when cooled.

Variations

Experiment with various flavorings: chocolate, raspberry, banana, poached fruit, dates, desserts wines, orange or lemon rind, coconut cream, nutmeg, cinnamon, and ground ginger.

I Yam What I Yam Sweet Potato Pie

Ingredients

- One 9-inch pie crust
- 3 pounds of sweet potatoes (bright orange)
- 4-6 tablespoons of butter
- 1/2-3/4 cup of sugar (to taste)
- 1 egg
- ½ cup of evaporated milk
- 1 teaspoon vanilla
- 1/2 teaspoon nutmeg (the secret ingredient)

Prepare a single 9-inch pie crust using cold ingredients. Preheat oven 425 degrees and bake three pounds of sweet potatoes/yams for approximately twenty-five minutes. Then prick the skins with a fork and continue baking at 350 degrees for twenty-five minutes or until done.

Scoop hot flesh of sweet potatoes into a large mixing bowl. Add butter, sugar, egg, and vanilla extract. Beat well with mixer or by hand for two minutes. Add evaporated milk and nutmeg. Pour into the pie shell. Bake pie at 350 degrees until pie crust is beautifully brown but not burnt. Serve room temperature.

Raw-Raw-Raw Chocolate Buttermilk Cake

This is a single-layer cake that can be formed into a bundt or spring foam cake pan. It is a simple yet noble sensation.

Ingredients

- 1 cup water
- 8 tablespoon butter (cut into pieces)
- 1/2 cup raw cacao powder or unsweetened cocoa powder
- 2 cups plain all-purpose flour, sifted
- 1 teaspoon baking soda (not powder)
- 1 1/2 cups sugar (caster or superfine)
- 2 eggs
- 1/2 cup buttermilk
- 1 teaspoon vanilla extract
- 1/2 teaspoon cinnamon (the secret ingredient)

Preheat oven to 350 degrees. Prepare cake pan (lightly greased and dusted with flour) with parchment/wax paper. In a sauce pan over medium heat, mix and melt water, butter, and cacao/cocoa powder. Meanwhile, measure and sift together flour, baking soda, and sugar. Whisk the cocoa/butter/water mixture with the dry ingredients. Add eggs, buttermilk, vanilla extract, and cinnamon. Whisk until dry elements disappear. Pour the entire mixture into your preferred baking dish. Bake forty to fifty minutes or until done when tested with a skewer or toothpick. Allow to cool, remove from baking dish, and dust with sifted confectioner's sugar as frosting. Any other icing diminishes the glory of the cake.

Afterword

Personal responsibility and genetic destiny determine the quality and quantity of one's life.
May you enjoy the blessings of health, fitness, and lean body.

About the Author

Carl Blake is a passionate eater and seeker of knowledge. His keenest interest is living life with simplicity and vitality. He has written and participated in public forums on a wide range of nutritional topics. Carl holds a doctor of musical arts degree in piano performance from Cornell University and is a two-time recipient of the Fulbright Scholar Award. Dr. Blake has traveled throughout the world teaching piano and performing at national and international venues to creditable critical acclaim.

Bibliography

Afrika, Llaila O. *African Holistic Health*. 2004.

Anderson, Nina, S.P.N., and Dr. Howard Peiper. *Low Carb and Beyond*. 2004.

Amen, Daniel G. *Change Your Brain, Change Your Body*. 2010.

Aziz, Michael, MD. *The Perfect Ten (Hormones) Diet*. 2010.

Braverman, Eric R. *The Healing Nutrients Within*. 2003 (revised).

Brazier, Brendan. *Thrive: The Vegan Nutrition Guide to Performance in Sports and Life*. 2007.

Cordain, Loren, PhD. *The Paleo Answer*. 2012.

   The Paleo Diet for Athletes. 2005.

Cousens, Gabriel, MD. *Rainbow Green Live-Foods Cuisine*. 2003.

Daoust, Joyce and Gene. *40-30-30 Fat Burning Nutrition*. 1996.

Davis, Brenda, RD, and Vesanto Melina, MS, RD. *Becoming Raw: The Essential Guide to Raw Vegan Diets*. 2010.

Davis, William, MD. *Wheat Belly*. 2011.

Delany, Brian M., and Lisa Walford. *The Longevity Diet*. 2010.

DeVany, Arthur. *Evolutionary Diet*. 2009.

Eramus, Udo. *Fats That Kill and Fats That Heal*. 1986.

Fallon, Sally. *Nourishing Traditions*. 2001.

Ferriss, Timothy. *The 4-Hour Body*. 2010.

Fossel, Michael, MD, PhD, Greta Blackburn, and Dave Woynarowski, MD. *The Immortality Edge*. 2011.

Fuhrmann, Joel, MD. *Super Immunity*. 2011.

Gedgaudas, Nora. *Primal Body, Primal Mind*. 2011.

Glassman, Keri. *The O2 Diet*. 2010.

Gundry, Steven, MD. *Dr. Gundry's Diet Evolution*. 2008.

Hofmekler, Ori. *Maximum Muscle: Minimum Fat*. 2008.

   Unlocking theMuscle Gene. 2011.

Hyman, Mark, MD. *Ultra-Metabolism: The Simple Plan for Automatic Weight Loss*. 2006.

Katz, Sandor Ellix. *Wild Fermentation: The Flavor, Nutrition, and Craft of Live-Culture Foods*. 2003.

Lauren, Mark with Joshua Clark. *You Are Your Own Gym*. 2011.

Loyd, Alexander with Ben Johnson. *The Healing Code*. 2010.

Mateljan, George. *The World's Healthiest Foods: Essential Guide*. 2007.

McGuff, Doug, MD, and John Little. *Body by Science*. 2009.

Minger, Denise. *Raw Food SOS*. http://rawfoodsos.com

Minich, Deanna M. *Chakra Food for Optimum Health*. 2009.

Murray, Michael, and Michael Lyon. *Hunger Free Forever*. 2007.

Pallardy, Pierr. *The Gut Instinct*. 2006.

Pollan, Michael. *Food Rules: An Eater's Manual*. 2009.

Portman, Robert, PhD, and John Ivy, PhD. *Hardwired for Fitness*. 2011

Reinagle, Monica. *The Inflammation Free Diet Plan*. 2006.

Rivera, Jairo Restrepo, and Sebastiao Pinheiro. *Agricultura Organica*. 2009.

Rose, Natalie. *Raw Food Life Force Energy*. 2007.

Rubin, Joshua. *Raw Truth: Transform Your Health With The Power Of Living Nutrients*. 2010.

Sears, Al, MD. *P.A.C.E. The 12-Minute Revolution*. 2010.

Shinya, Hiromi, MD. *The Enzyme Factor: Diet for the Future*. 2005.

Simopoulos, Artemis MD, and Jo Robinson. *The Omega Diet*. 1998.

Sisson, Mark. *Primal Blueprint*. 2010.

Somersall, PhD, MD, ed. *The Healing Power of 8 Sugars*. 2005.

Strunz, Ulrich, Dr. *Forever Young Fitness Drinks*. 2008.

Suarez, Frank. *The Power of Your Metabolism*. 2009.

Taubes, Gary. *Why We Get Fat and What To Do About It*. 2011.

USDA Dietary Guidelines. 2010.

Wolfe, David. *The Sunfood Diet Success System*. 2006.

Wood, Rebecca. *The Splendid Grain.* 1997.

Young, Robert PhD, and Shelley Redford Young. *The pH Miracle: Balance Your Diet, Reclaim Your Health.* 2002.
The pH Miracle for Weight Loss. 2006.